Poultry Production and Hatchery Management

Poultry Production *and* Hatchery Management

Dr. M.T. Banday, Professor, B.V.Sc.;M.V.Sc.; Ph.D.
Division of Livestock Production and Management
Faculty of Veterinary Sciences and Animal Husbandry
Srinagar, SKUAST-Kashmir (J&K)

Dr. S. Adil, Assistant Professor, B.V.Sc; M.V.Sc
Division of Livestock Production and Management
Faculty of Veterinary Sciences and Animal Husbandry
Srinagar, SKUAST-Kashmir (J&K)

SSPH

SATISH SERIAL PUBLISHING HOUSE
403, Express Tower, Commercial Complex
Azadpur, Delhi-110033 (India)
Phone : 011-27672852, Fax : 91-11-27672046
e-mail : info@satishserial.com, hkjain1975@yahoo.com
Website : www.satishserial.com

Published by :

SATISH SERIAL PUBLISHING HOUSE

403, Express Tower, Commercial Complex, Azadpur, Delhi-110033 (INDIA)
Phone : 011-27672852 Fax : 91-11-27672046
E-mail : info@satishserial.com, hkjain1975@yahoo.com

ISBN 978-93-88020-31-2

Composed, Designed & Printed in India

Preface

Poultry farming in India was a backyard venture almost upto 1960. Indigenous Poultry which are hardy but poor in growth and productivity were used for the production of eggs and meat. Lack of interest in poultry improvement was due to low productivity of indigenous birds, low eggs and meat, inadequate knowledge of husbandry practices prejudices against raising of chicken and consumption of poultry egg and meat.

During last four decades the entire scenario of poultry farming in the country has change. It is now recognised and scientifically based industry and a potential to fight poverty and malnutrition. Thousands of Poultry farms, both small and large have come up all over the country and indigenous desi birds have given way to highly specialised layers and broilers. A network of hatcheries has been established in public and private sectors to supply quality commercial hybrid chicks.

Today, India ranks 4th in egg production and 19th in broiler production in the world. The growth rate for eggs and broiler production has been as high as 10 and 15 per cent respectively. Undoubtedly, what has been achieved is quite impressive. However, with globalisation of world trade, there is greater need to promote export-oriented poultry eggs and meat in the country.

In this context, a comprehensive book on poultry production and hatchery management has been written to fulfill a well and badly felt need of an elaborately covered topics which can cater the need of students, researchers, teachers and people affiliated with poultry and hatchers industry.

We are sure that this book would act as a guide to one and all in poultry sector for their individual and industrial development as it would make them aware to what extent they can grow by crossing the initial hurdles.

Last but not the least we are indebted to the poultry farmers of this country who are the real heroes for bringing the poultry industry on global map.

Authors

Contents

Chapter **1**

Introduction to Poultry Farming

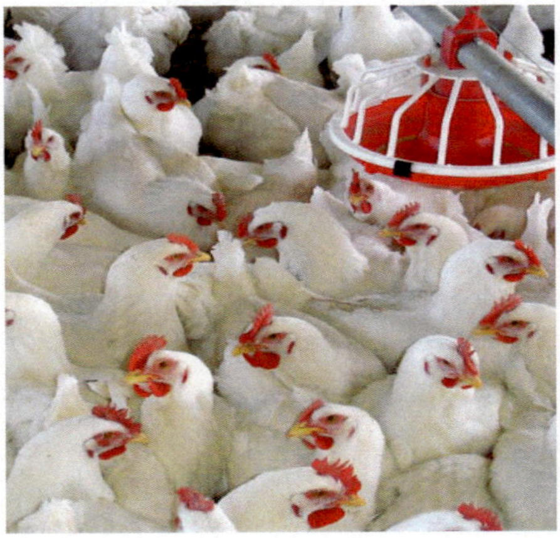

The term 'poultry' includes a number of avian species, such as chickens, ducks, turkey, quail, geese and guinea fowl domesticated for economic purposes. These adapt well under a wide range of agro climatic conditions and can successfully be raised, if proper management and nutritional requirements are provided. Chicken, ducks and quails are kept for production of both eggs and meat while turkey, guinea -fowl and geese are reared essentially for meat. The most common and widely used poultry birds in the world are chicken which may be either meat type birds called broiler chicken raised for meat production or egg type chicken called layer meant for egg production.

Poultry has a crucial place in India as the eggs and chicken meat are important and rich sources of protein, vitamins and minerals. Poultry also provides rich organic manure and is an important source of income and employment to millions of farmers and other persons engaged in allied activities in the poultry industry.

Poultry is one of the fastest growing segments of the agricultural sector in India with around eight per cent growth rate per annum. The poultry sector in India has undergone a paradigm shift in structure and operation which has been its transformation from a mere backyard activity into a major commercial agri based industry over a period of four decades. The constant efforts in upgradation, modification and application of new technologies paved the way for the multifold and multifaceted growth in poultry and allied sectors. The development is not only in size but also in productivity, sophistication and quality. Development of high yielding layer (310340 eggs) and broiler (2.4-2.6 kg at 6 wks) varieties together with standardized package of practices on nutrition, housing, management and disease control have contributed to spectacular growth rates in egg (4-6% per annum) and broiler production (8-10% per annum) in India during the last 40 years. The annual per capita availability also increased to 60 eggs and 2.5 Kg of meat, consistently with increase in productivity. However, it is far below the recommended level of consumption of 180 eggs and 10.8 kg poultry meat per person per annum by Indian Council Medical Research. This transformation has involved sizeable expansions and investments in breeding, hatching, rearing and processing. India is one of the few countries in the world that has put into place a sustained Specific Pathogen Free (SPF) egg production project. Indian poultry industry has emerged as one of the fastest growing segments of the agriculture sector today in India. As the production of agriculture crops is rising @ 2.5% per annum, the production of eggs has been rising @ 5.5% and broilers @11.44% per annum.

The growth of the poultry sector in India is also marked by an increase in the size of the poultry farm. In earlier years broiler farms had produced on average a few hundred birds (200-500 chicks) per cycle. Today units with fewer than 5,000 birds are becoming rare, and units with 5,000 to 50,000 birds per week cycle are common. Similarly, in layer farms, units with a flock size of 10,000 to 50,000 birds have become common. Small units are probably finding themselves at a disadvantage because of high feed and transport costs, expensive vaccines, and veterinary care services and the non-availability of credit. Some small units are reported to be shifting from layer to broiler production because output in broiler units can be realized in six weeks.

The structure of India's poultry industry varies from region to region. While independent and relatively small-scale producers account for the bulk of production, integrated large-scale producers account for a growing share of output in some regions. Integrators include large regional farms that incorporate all aspects of production, including the raising of grandparent and parent flocks, rearing DOCs, contracting production, compounding feed, providing veterinary services, and wholesaling. The southern region account for about 57 per cent of the country's egg production, the eastern and central regions of India account for about 17 per cent, the northern and western regions contribute 26% egg production.

Current scenario

India ranks 3rd in egg production and 7th in chicken meat production in the world. About 83 billion eggs are produced from 260 million layers and 3.4 million tons of poultry meat is produced from 3000 million broilers per annum in India. The Poultry Industry is contributing about Rs.70,000/crores to the national GDP and providing employment to more than 4 million people either directly or indirectly. About 2-2.5 million tons of poultry litter, a valuable organic fertilizer, is produced as a by-product every year. The poultry industry is concentrated in certain pockets of the country. The State of Andhra Pradesh, Telangana, Tamil Nadu lead the country followed by Maharashtra, Punjab and West Bengal.

The popularity of poultry meat is on the rise during the last two decades. It is presently accounting for about 45% of the total meat consumed and is the most popular meat from any single livestock species. Chicken dominates the poultry production in India with nearly 95% of the total egg production and the rest is contributed by ducks and others. Majority of ducks are found in certain states on the eastern and southern coast like West Bengal, Assam, Odisha, Kerala, Andhra Pradesh, Tamil Nadu, etc. Other species like turkeys, guinea fowls, ostriches, emus, etc. are reared only in small numbers in areas having specific market demand. India is the home for many breeds of native chicken like Aseel, KadakNath, Tellicherry, Haringhata Black, Nicobari, Danki, etc., which are still popular among the rural and tribal areas for backyard/ free range farming. For the commercial farming, high yielding crosses developed and supplied by the private sector like Babcock, Bovans (egg type) and Cobb, Ross, Hubbard (meat type) are being used. The crosses developed under the public sector like Krishilayer, Krishibro (multicoloured broiler, etc.) are popular in certain areas.

Availability of eggs is highly non-uniform in different parts of the country primarily due to wide variation in the production levels. Much of the eggs produced are consumed by the urban population while the rural and tribal areas have little access to the eggs and meat produced from the industrial sources and the availability is very low. In spite of rapid growth, the poultry industry suffered many setbacks in recent times due to rising cost of feed, emergence of new or re-emerging of existing diseases, fluctuating market price of egg and broilers, etc. which need to be addressed to make the poultry sector as a sustainable enterprise.

Table 1: Egg production and per capita availability in India

Year	Egg (Million numbers)	Human Population (Million numbers)	Per Capita Availability (Numbers / Head / Annum)
1950-51	1832	359	5
1960-61	2881	434	7
1968-69	5300	518	10
1980-81	10060	679	15
1990-91	21101	839	25
2000-01	36632	1019	36
2010-11	63024	1186	53
2015-16	83640	1230	68

Table 2: Time line with major milestones of Indian egg production

Year	Milestones
1950-51	Backyard poultry with native breeds and low egg production by dual purpose birds.
1955	Hybrid White Leg Horn (WLH) introduced
1965	Key Village Scheme (KVS)
1970	All India Coordinated Research Project (AICRP) on Egg
1975	Cage rearing of layers
1982	National Egg Coordination Committee (NECC), Support from banks, Establishment of feed and pharmaceutical industries.
1995	High platform cages, Vertical integration, Corporate tendency
2000	Automation in feeding, egg collection, environmental controlled housing, exports, egg powder production plants.
2010	High capacity farms with low margins.

Reasons for Improved Egg Production and Productivity Differences

The reasons for increased productivity of commercial hybrid layers over the years are due to several reasons. Some of them are:

1. Strong private sector participation.
2. Investments by public & private sectors in poultry sector.
3. Improvements in genetic potential of poultry.
4. Advances in feeding technology like least cost formulation, pelleted feeding, feed additives, provision of fed by integrators, feed analytical laboratories for quality control, etc.
5. Advances in healthcare like vaccines and medication.
6. Adoption of bio-security measures – water sanitation, restricted entry of personnel into farms, dead bird disposal, etc.
7. Improved breeder management and chick quality.

The genetic potential of commercial layer chicks being supplied by public and private institutions is almost same. However, the productivity varies in different parts of the country due to:

1. Influence of climatic conditions and weather.
2. Availability of inputs and services.
3. Dissimilar entrepreneurial nurture of farmers.
4. Great variation in management practices.
5. Economy of scale in production.

Andhra Pradesh is leading state in egg production followed by Tamil Nadu, Maharashtra, West Bengal, Haryana and Punjab, which accounts for 80 % of eggs produced in India.

For table eggs, National Egg Coordination Committee (NECC) fixes and publishes daily prices for each of the major production and consumption centres.

Polutry meat production in india

India is the 9th largest producer of poultry meat in the world. Poultry meat production has increased from 0.069 million tonnes in 1961 to 3.04 million tonnes in 2014-15. The per capita availability of poultry meat is 2.50 kg as against recommended level of 11 kg of meat per annum.

Table 3: Trends in poultry meat production in India ('000 tonnes)

Year	Poultry Meat Production	Per capita Availability of Poultry Meat (Kg)
1980	179	0.266
1990	412	0.498
2000	980	0.820
2005	1900	1.300
2010	2337	2.150
2015	3402	2.50

Table 4: Time line with major milestones of Indian poultry meat production

Year	Milestones
1962	Meat type strains imported from Israel
1970	All India Coordinated Research Projects (AICRP)
1974	Import of Cobb strain
1980	Entry of private sector (Cobb + Venkateswara), Pureline broiler stock, Multiple batch farms, Market in urban areas.
1995	Introduction of contract broiler farming, All -in – all -out batches, Rural based production and urban marketing, Improved bio-security
2000	Growth of contract broiler farming, Hatcheries, Feed mills, Feed additives
2010	High capacity farms with low margins, Entry of broiler breeding giants, Growth performance matching with world standards –2.2 kg at 37 days with 1.6 Feed Conversion Ratio.

Reasons for Improved Poultry Meat Production

The reasons for improved poultry meat production are:

1. Private sector partnerships through contract broiler farming.
2. Modernization of production practices
3. Import of Pure lines/ grandparent stock.
4. Least cost feed formulation.
5. Vaccines against major diseases.
6. Availability of support services.
7. Improved quality breeder management.
8. Developments in poultry processing.

The contract broiler farming system has played a major role in the spectacular growth especially in Southern and Western states with almost 75 % of broiler meat being produced under contract farming. During the last three decades, there have been major changes in structure, size and number of broiler farms. Now a typical broiler farmer raises 5000 to 50000 for a weekly cycle compared to few hundred in 1990s. Due to modernization of production and management practices, the body weight which was achieved at 8 weeks of age during the 1980s is now realized in 35 to 40 days of age.

The leading states in poultry meat production are :

1. Telangana (Hyderabad- Vijayawada belt)
2. Tamil Nadu (Coimbatore – Salem belt)
3. Maharashtra (Pune- Nasik- Mumbai belt)
4. Haryana (Gurgaon- Yamunanagar belt)

The Broiler Coordination Committee, Coimbatore sets the broiler prices for different regions and price varies daily. These rates are considered the benchmark rate for broilers in India.

❑❑❑

Chapter 2

Biology of Chicken

Nomenclature

The biology of domestic fowl is closely related to the biology of other birds. Knowing some of the features of avian biology can aid in understanding the factors that influence the ability of chicken to lay eggs, grow rapidly and serve as an efficient source of human food.

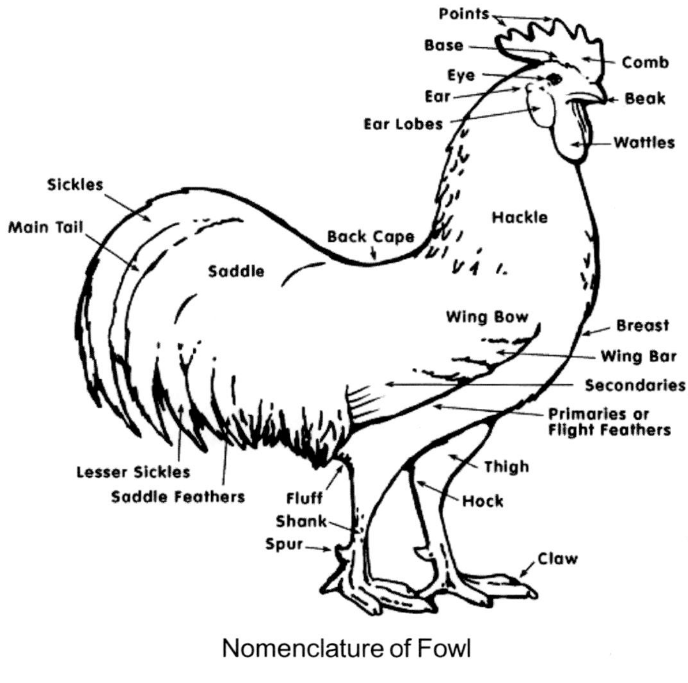

Nomenclature of Fowl

Skeletal System

The skeletal system of fowl is compact, light in weight and very strong. The vertebrae of the neck and the tail are movable but the body of chicken has only one movable vertebrae. The body of the vertebrae are fused into rigid structures. Many bones of the birds are pneumatic i.e. they are hollow and are connected to the respiratory system. Many bones contain a unique type of bone called medullary bone. This bone provides a readily available source of calcium for egg shell formation when calcium intake is low. Nearly 12% of the total bone of a mature hen may be medullary bone.

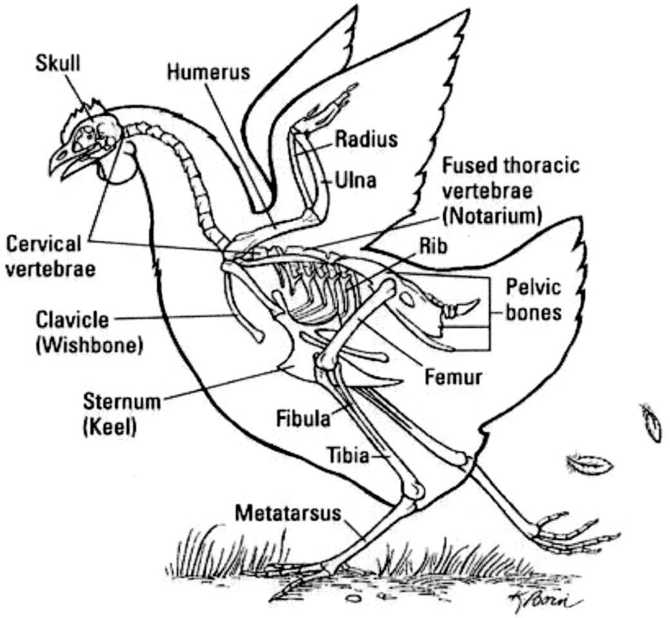

Skeletal system of fowl

Muscular System

Three principal types or muscles are present in chicken. They are smooth muscle, cardiac muscle and skeletal muscle. The breast, thigh and leg muscles are the most prominent muscle in the body of the bird. Because of the adaptation of birds to flight, the breast muscles are large and well-developed. They contribute one by twelfth of the entire body weights of birds.

Respiratory System

The respiratory system consists of the lungs, the passage leading to the lungs and the air sacs. The lungs are closely attached to the ribs in the upper portion of the thoracic cavity. The lungs are rather rigid structures which expand and contract relatively little during respiration. It is primarily change in pressure within air sacs that cause air to pass into and out of the lungs. The chicken has 4 pairs of air sacs, ranging in position from the neck to the abdomen, with a single medium sac located in the cavity of the thorax. These sacs open into the lungs and communicate with the pneumatic bones of the body. The air sacs are delicate, thin walled structures.

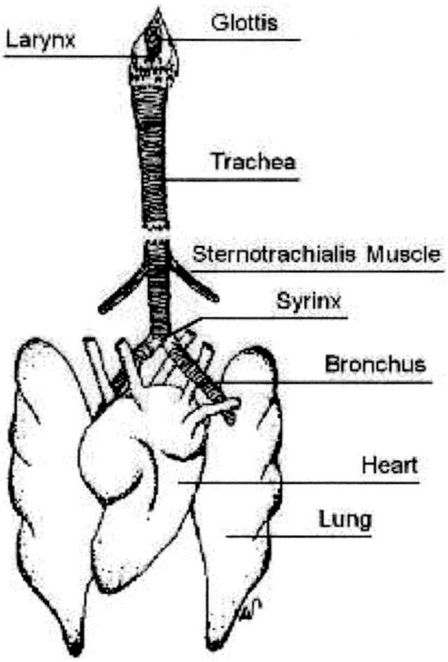

Respiratory system of chicken

The voice of the fowl is produced in the syrinx or lower larynx, located where the trachea divides into two bronchi. The syrinx is the only part of the respiratory tract that is capable of producing sound, upper larynx serves to modulate the voice. The normal hen does not crow because she lacks the physiological incentive to do so.

The Skin

Chicken has a relatively thin skin which is free of secretary glands. The only exception is the uropygial or oil gland (Preen gland), which is found on the upper portion of the tail. Numerous specialized structures are associated with the skin, such as the comb; wattles are particularly associated with gonad development and secretion of the sex hormones.

Skin colour depends on combination of pigments in the upper and lower of skin. Yellow skin and shanks are due to carotenoid pigments of dietary origin in the epidermis (upper layer) along with a absence of melanic pigment. Black and its variations are caused by the presence of melanic pigment in the epidermis. The darkest shank occurs when melanic pigment is present in both the dermis (lower layer) and the epidermis. White shank results from the complete absence of both types of pigments.

Feathers : The feathers are epidermal structures. They help to protect the birds from external injuries. Keep body warm and help in flight. Feathers are arranged in rows within definite tract (pterylae) in the skin of poultry. The tracts are separated by non-feathered spaces (apteria). Feathers can be divided into three types:

a) Plumules : Are small downy feathers covered by contour feathers in adult birds. They provide insulation and help to retain body heat.

b) Fitoplumes : Are intermediate types of feathers. They are hair like structures which remain after bird has been plucked.

c) Contour feathers : Include all other feathers covering the body of the bird e.g., flight feathers of wing and tail, the covert feathers which furrow over the base of the flight feathers and contour feathers which streamline the body.

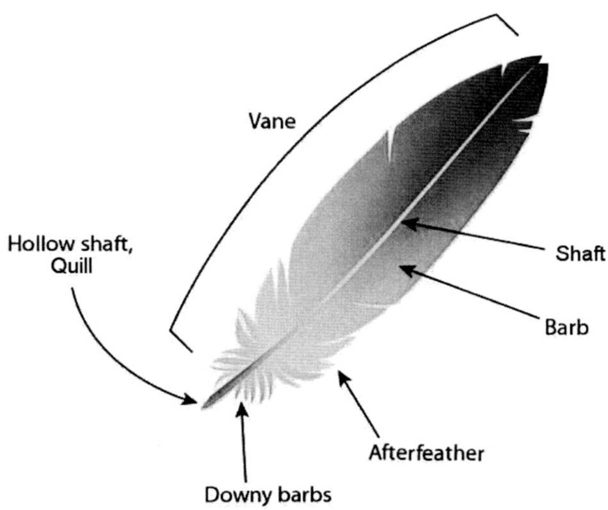

Structure of a feather

The parts of a typical contour feather are shafts; the lover part of the shaft is hallow and is called as the joint of quill and shaft, there are fluffy filaments called after shaft, extending on either sides of the shaft, are many parallel branches called barbs, the barbs in turn have branches known s barbules, the barbules have tiny hooks, the barbicels which serve to hold the parts of the feather solidly together.

Circulatory System

The chicken has a four chambered heart, two atria and two ventricles. The blood of a chicken makes up about 8% of the body weight in chicks of one to two weeks of age and about 6% of weight of a mature hen. The heart rate of a mature white leghorn is about 350 beats per minute. Heavy breeds have a lower heart rate averaging about 250 beats per minute.

Circulatory system of chicken

The major functions of blood are:

a) They help in the transportation of oxygen and carbon dioxide.

b) They help in the transportation of nutrients to body cells.

c) They help in temperature regulation.

d) They help in transportation of important metabolites, hormones and waste products to appropriate places in the body.

Excretory System

The excretion of water and metabolic wastes occurs largely through the kidneys. The avian kidney is rather large elongated organs located tightly against the top of the abdominal cavity closely associated with backbone. Each kidney is divided into three separate readily visible lobes. The kidney is made up of many small tubules or nephrons which are the main functional features of the kidney. Water and compounds conserved by the body are largely reabsorbed while waste products to be eliminated are excreted in the urine. The kidney has a key role in regulating acid-base balance and maintaining osmotic balance of body fluids. Chicken urine is yellowish fluid containing a white pasty substance (whitecap) that is largely uric acid. This material gives bird droppings their characteristic white appearance. Uric acid is the end product of protein metabolism in birds and is water insoluble compound. The urine passes out of the kidney through the ureters which end in the cloaca. This is a chamber common to the digestive, urinary and reproductive passages which open externally at the vent.

Male Reproductive System

The male reproductive system of poultry is extremely simple, consisting of two testes, each having an epididymis and vas deferens that lead to the copulatory organ. The male bird is unique among domestic animals in that the testes are located along the back bone within the abdominal cavity. Birds have evolved a mechanism, in which intra-abdominal testes are fully functional. The copulatory apparatus of chicken consists of two papillae and a rudimentary copulatory organ that is located at the vent.

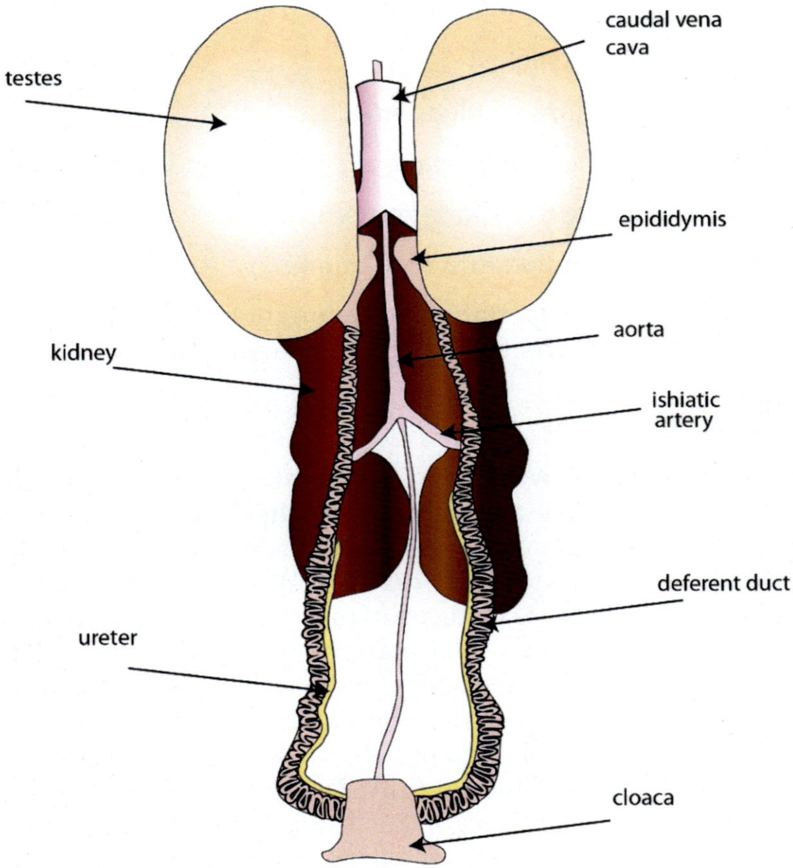

Urinary and reproductive system of male chicken

Female Reproductive System

The female reproductive system comprises of an **ovary** and **oviduct**. The oviduct is further classified into infundibulum, magnum, isthumus, uterus and vagina. In all the birds, only the left ovary and oviduct is functional while those on right side are rudimentary.

Ovary looks like a cluster of grapes is located anterior to kidneys in dorsal part of abdominal cavity. It contains yellowish spherical bodies called yolks or ova in different stages of development. An ovary may have 900-3500 follicles.

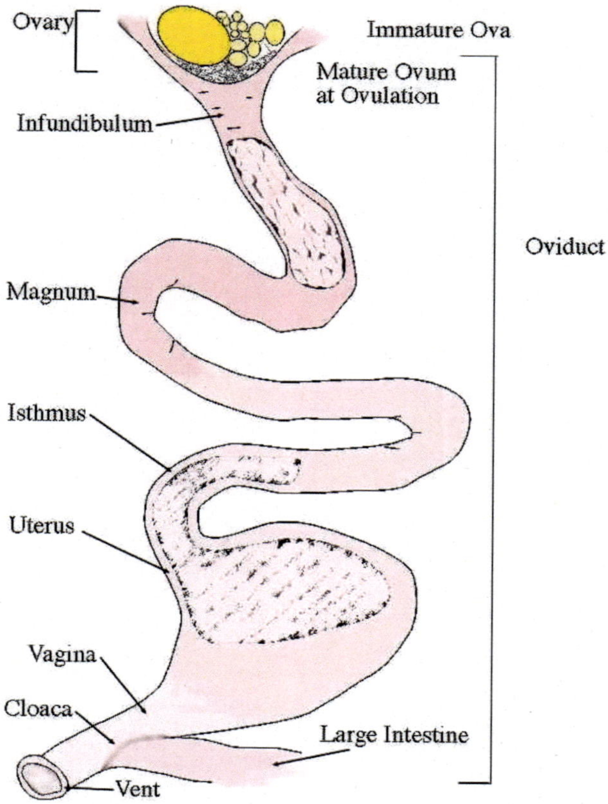

Female reproductive system of chicken

Depending upon the laying stage of hen, its weight may vary from 3-52 g.

- Infundibulum is 8-10 cm long funnel shaped structure.

- Magnum measures 33-36 cm and is the largest segment of the oviduct.
- Isthumus is about 10 cm long section of the oviduct
- Uterus is about 10 cm in length also known as shell gland.
- Vagina is about 5 cm long part of oviduct that opens into cloaca.

Chapter 3

Egg Formation and Egg Quality

The Structure of an Egg

An egg consists of various parts viz. cuticle, shell, air cell and inner and outer shell membranes, outer thin albumen, inner thick albumen, chalazae, yolk membrane, germinal disk, yolk, and chalaziferous albumen.

The shell has an outer coating called the **cuticle.** The cuticle acts as a barrier to keep bacteria from entering the egg and thus, provides a defense against various invading bacteria. If the eggs are mechanically washed, cuticle gets removed from the eggs.

The **shell** has almost 8,000 tiny pores and is made almost entirely of calcium. The rate of calcium deposition during egg shell formation and the amount of time egg spends in the uterus determines its thickness. The shell prevents various substances from entering the egg but is semi-permeable and allows the gaseous exchange.

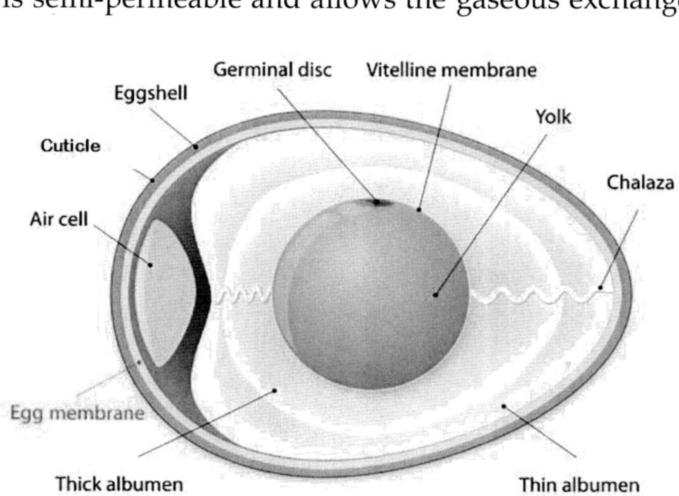

Structure of an egg

When the egg is laid and the contents of the egg cool down, an **air space** gets formed. It gets formed at the larger end, usually between the outer and inner membranes at the egg. With the age of egg, air enters in to the egg and moisture and carbon dioxide leave the egg through pores and this result in the larger air cells.

The inner and outer shell membranes are present immediately inside the shell surrounding the egg white. These are made partly of keratin and just like cuticle provide an efficient defense against invasive bacteria.

The outer thin albumen lies next to the shell membrane and is a narrow fluid layer. It is located farthest from the yolk.

The inner thick white (chalaziferous layer) is located nearest to the yolk and is a dense, matted, fibrous capsule of albumen. It is rich source of protein and riboflavin.

Chalazae serve to keep the yolk incenter and are twisted in opposite directions. The prominence of chalazae indicates the more freshness of egg.

Yolk membrane encloses the egg yolk.

Germinal disk is a small, white circular spot on the surface of the yolk and is a spot where the sperm enters the egg. From germinal disk, embryo develops.

Yolk is yellow in colour and is a major source of fat, cholesterol, vitamins, minerals, and good source of proteins.

Chalaziferous albumen is present around the membrane of the yolk and is a dense fibrous capsule of albumen.

Chemical Composition of Eggs

Egg has three main parts viz. the shell, the egg white and the egg yolk.

In shell calcite crystals are embedded in a matrix of proteins and polysaccharide complex. Inside the shell there is a viscous colourless liquid known as egg white which accounts for about 58% of the total egg weight. The chief constituents of egg white besides water are proteins. Different types of proteins are present in egg white viz. ovalbumin, conalbumin, ovamucoid, ovomucin, lysozyme, avidin, ovoglobulin and ovoinhibitor. Ovalbumin is the main protein of egg weight and constitutes about 55% of the total proteins of egg white. Yolk is mainly rich in fats (32.5%).

Table 1: Chemical composition of an egg

Component	Egg with shell	Yolk & Albumen	Yolk	Albumen
Water (%)	65.6	73.6	48.7	87.9
Protein (%)	12.1	12.8	16.6	10.6
Lipids (%)	10.5	11.8	32.6	Traces
Carbohydrates (%)	0.9	1.0	1.0	0.9
Minerals (%)	10.9	0.8	1.10	0.6

Egg protein is unique in that it contains all of the 8 amino acids considered essential for growth and maintenance of body tissues. It is therefore regarded as a balanced protein which when added to other foods of unbalanced protein, serves to complement their nutritive value.

Egg fat is in an emulsifying form, readily digestible not only by adults but even by infants, as young as 3 months old. Egg fat is rich in phosphorus and is essential fatty acid. It is also the carrier of much of the egg's vitamin content. The iron content of egg is relatively high in comparison to other foods and is in a readily available form. Egg contains a number of other minerals in useful amount as shown below:

Table 2: Nutrient percent in an egg

Nutrient	One egg contains	% of daily requirement for an average adult supplied by an egg
Protein	6.7 g	10
Calorie	90.0	2-3
Calcium	0.3 g	5
Phosphorus	0.11 g	10
Vitamin A	200-800 I.U.	4-16
Vitamin D	10-50 I.U.	2-12
Thiamine (B1)	60-120 mcg	1-5
Riboflavin	100-500 mcg	5-23
Niacin	760 mcg	5-11

Egg Formation

Depending on breed and age, hens are at peak production during their first few years of life, and as they get older, total egg production and its quality decreases. The ovary contains the developing follicles like a bunch of grapes.

Once the ovary releases ovum, it is engulfed by the infundibulum, at the proximal end of the oviduct. Thereafter, the ovum is propelled distally through the oviduct. If the male chicken is present, the fertilization of the ovum takes place in the infundibulum. Initially the Chalaza appears as fine filaments while the ovum is in the infundibulum. From here the egg moves to the infandibulum and it takes less than 30 minutes.

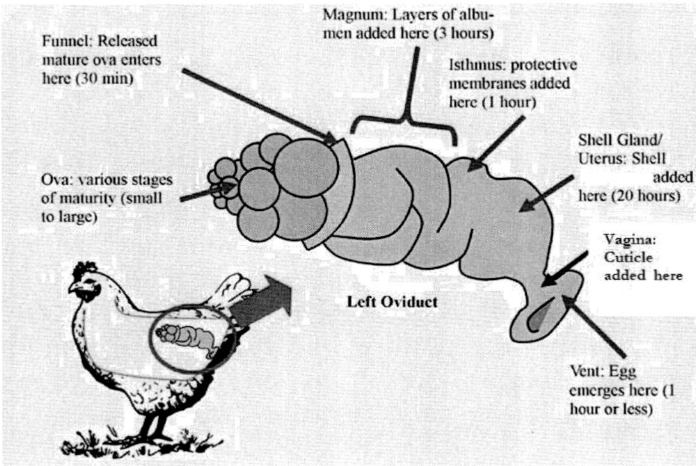

Formation of chicken egg

In the magnum, the egg gets covered with a coating of albumen (egg white) in about 3 hours. From here the egg moves to the Isthmus.

In the isthmus, shell membranes are deposited around the egg. This is a fast process taking approximately 1 hour. Thereafter, the egg moves to the uterus.

In the uterus the outer shell and shell pigments are deposited. The egg spends the highest period of time (approximately 20 hours) in the uterus region. The shell is mainly composed composed of calcium carbonate which is extracted from partly from the hen's own body stores of calcium (47%) and dietary calcium (53%). So, it is important that hen's diet is rich in calcium.

In the vagina, a protective shell coating called the cuticle (bloom) gets deposited around the egg just prior to laying. The cuticle protects the egg from bacterial invasion during its passage through the cloaca.

The total time taken for egg formation is approximately 25 hours.

Egg Quality

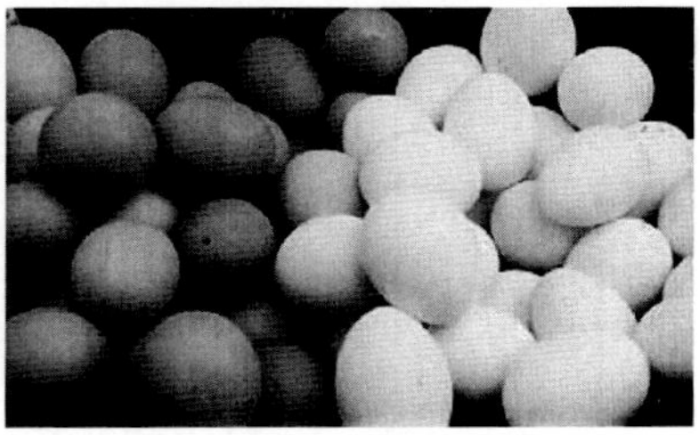

Quality may be regarded as the inherent properties of a product which determines its degree of excellence. This definition if "Quality" applies to eggs. In simple words, quality of eggs may be judged on the basis of characteristics which the consumer prefers and is willing to pay for. Although, in a general sense, the quality of an egg may be considered under organoleptic (sensory), nutrition, functional and sanitary aspects, the consumer is the final judge of what constitutes quality. Thus, the choice and opinion of consumers, is of great consequence in recognising egg quality and for adoption of quality standards in the marketing of eggs. Broadly egg quality may be considered under:-

A. External quality

B. Internal quality

A. External Quality of Eggs

1. Egg shape and colour
2. Size or weight of the egg
3. Shell quality
4. Cleanliness

1. Egg shape and colour

An ideal shape of egg is oval or ovate, with one end larger than the other, giving it a tapered appearance. While most eggs are usually normal shaped, slight departure in the shape of eggs does not constitute a major defect. Even prescribed at and standards for egg quality allow eggs to be of slightly abnormal shape. However, occasionally wide variations in the shape of eggs are encounted such as off-shape, misshapen eggs, etc. which constitute a major abnormality because of lowered eye appeal and greater risk of breakages in the market channels.

Colour of egg shells is of relatively less importance. The egg trade recognises only two colours i) The white shelled eggs and ii) the brown shed eggs. The brownish shade may vary from being dark to light brown in colour. The brown colour of eggs, is a typical characteristic of some breeds of hens (mostly American and English classes or their crosses) that is, genetically controlled. Sometimes, the expression "coloured" or tinted eggs are used to donate the brown eggs. Regardless of the colour, uniformity in colour of a given lot is desirable.

2. Size or weight of the egg

Size of the egg is measured by its weight. It is an important external quality characteristic and is also considered in the grading of eggs. An average or acceptable egg size may vary around 55g. However, consumers generally prefer eggs that are bigger in size and in well organised markets, larger eggs carry a premium price. Occasionally excessively large eggs, double yolk eggs or excessively small (pullet eggs) may be observed. This is not constitute desirable size characteristics as such eggs may be more prone to breakages specially when packed and shipped or may have lowered consumer acceptance (small sized eggs), when eggs are packed in egg trays/egg cartons/ egg cases, etc. Uniformity of size in a given lot should receive proper attention.

3. Shell Quality

The shell of high quality eggs sound and strong. More precisely shell quality may be considered under such standards like i) shell prosity ii) shell thickness iii) shell strength iv) shell per cent, etc. However, in the marketing of eggs, shell quality is referred to in terms of soundness eggs with poor shell quality or those having weak shells may break and spoils other eggs while handling or in transit, this external quality characteristic assumes considerable importance. Also because poor shell quality renders eggs liable to greater and rapid internal quality losses.

4. Cleanliness

Eggs should have a clean appearance; this makes them look more attractive and hygienic, and reduces the risk of microbiological contamination from the surface to the contents. Poultry producers should therefore pay greater attention to the production of naturally clean (nest-clean) eggs through sound, management practices. Clean eggs have butter keeping quality. Even though dirty eggs can be cleaned or washed (not in plain water but according to acceptable scientific procedures), their storage life become greatly reduced.

A clean egg must be free from stains, such as dirt, excreta, blood, yolk material or any other type of extraneous material adhering to it. However, eggs having small specks or attains which do not make it un-attractive are considered practically clean and permitted even where grading is carried out.

B. Internal Quality of Eggs

The internal quality of table eggs may include the following:

1. Size and position of air cell
2. Albumen condition
3. Yolk shape and colour
4. Freedom from defects and
5. Flavour, etc.

1. Size and position of Air cells

The air cell, located at the broad and of the egg should be small. It usually has a depth of about 4 mm. In good quality egg, while it may be comparatively larger in eggs of somewhat poor quality. The air cell size gives an indication of the extent of evaporation from eggs. Although air cell depth can be precisely measured (by using and Air cell gauge), in common practice a visual judgment is used at candling time in assessing the size of the air cell. In high quality eggs, the air cell is not only small, practically regular but maintains almost a fixed position with a clear outline. It does not tend to move when rotated at the candling light. Air cell defects like freely moving air cell, bubbly air cell which generally arise from rough handling tend to lower egg quality. Air cell defects are undesirable.

2. Albumen condition

In a normal and high quality egg, the albumen is firm and viscous with greater percentage of thick albumen. Thus, albumen quality can be indicated by the amount and height of thick albumen. Sometimes other measures like thick albumen and thin albumen, thin albumen diameter, percentage of thick and thin albumen, etc. have been used as measures of albumen condition. However, the height of thick albumen itself can give a fair idea of albumen condition. This can easily be ascertained by actually measuring the height of the thick albumen from an opened egg or even by holding the egg contents on a flat plate at eye level and nothing how high thick albumen appears. As more reliable measures of albumen quality, height of thick albumen itself or the ratio of height to the width of the thick albumen is used. The latter is called albumen index. Sometimes, especially in scientific studies a certain relationship is used where in the height of the thick albumen adjusted to the weight of the egg is employed to determine albumen quality. This measure is called as Haugh Unit (H.U) score, anmed after its originator Dr. R.R. haugh of the U.S.A . Higher Haugh Unit Scores indicates better egg (albumen) quality.

3. Yolk shape and colour

In high quality fresh eggs, the yolk is spherical in shape (but not perfectly round) and tends to be in the centre of the egg that is broken open and stands well above the surrounding thick albumen with a characteristic golden yellow appealing colour. However, both the shape and colour are subject to variation. This difference in yolk colour is due to differences in the xanthophylls content. A desirable yolk colour varies widely depending upon individual consumers. Standards based on visual comparison or yolk pigment assays are availble for colour evaluation. Eggs of good quality have uniform golden yellow yolk colour and its appearance can be regulated through proper feeding programmes for obtaining maximum consumer satisfaction.

As the egg gets older, that is, ages" there is actually passage of water from the albumen to the yolk which results in the yolk losing its normal shape and becoming flat; causing poor quality. In measuring yolk quality, the height and width of the yolk are determined and the ratio of height to the width (yolk height divided by mean yolk diameter) is calculated. This is referred to as yolk index.

4. Freedom from Defects

High quality eggs should be free from such defects as blood spots, meat spots, rots or other showing evidence of germ development or partially developed embryos, etc. Eggs that have become specified due to presence of bacteria or moulds are usually called as rots. All rots are unfit for human consumption. It is considered a serious defect if the vetelline membrane is broken, allowing the white to mix with the yolk. Such eggs are called addled eggs.

i) Blood spots : Blood spots in eggs constitute a fairly common defect. A blood spot is believed to arise from the rupture of a small blood vessel in the follicle while the yolk is being formed. The result is that a small clot of blood is enclosed within the egg, usually on the surface of the yolk. They appear as a red dark spot or streak on the yolk. They appear vary greatly in size, shape and frequency. It is commonly assumed that from 2 to 4 percent of all chicken eggs, contain blood spots which are invariably found on the yolk. Blood spots are very common in the eggs of heavy breeds and also show seasonal variation. Blood spots in the eggs lower the consumer acceptance; hence such eggs containing detectable blood spots should not be marketed. Selective breeding programmes and an adequacy of vitamin A and even K in poultry feeds have been shown to keep and incidence of these inclusions within lower and tolerable limits.

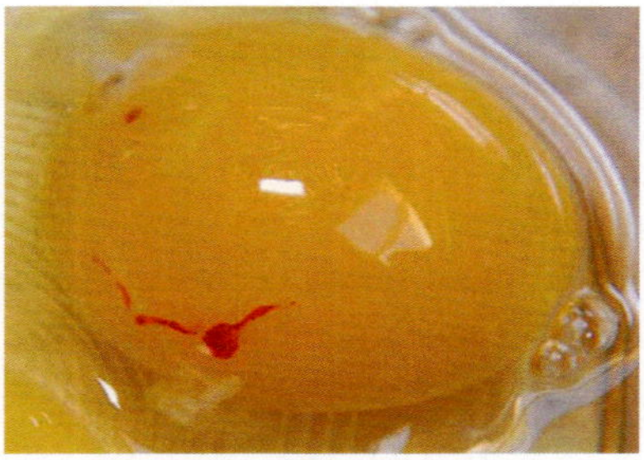

Blood spots

ii) Meat spots : A second common internal defect or inclusion is meat spots. These are usually light, brown or liver like in colour, usually freely floating on the albumen and sometimes on the yolk. Meat spots were formally thought to consist of tissues sloughed off from the walls of oviduct which become included with the egg. Recent observations, however, indicate that they seem to be actually blood spots which have undergone a certain amount of degenerative, chemical or pigmentry changes to appear differently. Both blood and meat spots may be identified during candling or in the opened eggs. All spots having the appearance of fresh blood are considered as blood spots, while the others are regarded as meat spots. Light coloured meat spots

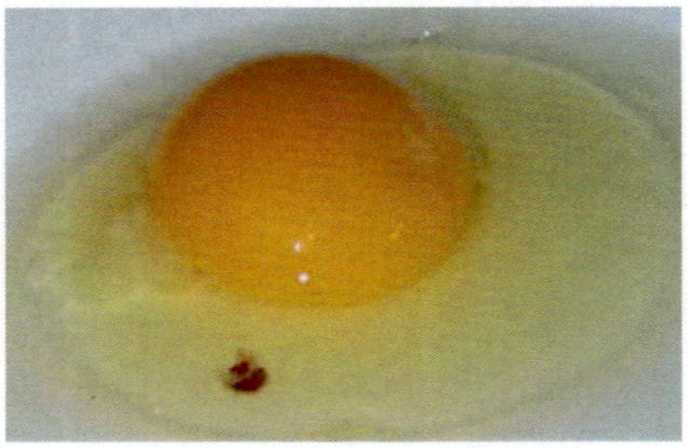

Meat spots

and pin-point blood spots are the more common and more difficult to detect egg inclusions. Regardless of their orgin, the presence of blood or meat spots in eggs renders them unfit for consumption.

5. **Flavour**

Flavour has been defined as dual sensory responses based on taste and small, that is, oral and nasal senses. Eggs are characterised by particular likeable flavour. However, under some conditions eggs may exhibit undesirable flavours, e.g., earthy odours, must flavour, rishy flavours, etc. Eggs with off odours or undesirable flavours lower acceptability for human consumption or result in their becoming inedible.

Factors Affecting Egg Quality and Quality Determination

I. Quality of fresh eggs

Eggs are regarded as an item of human food almost unsurpassed in nutritive excellence. The internal quality of the egg is at its best when freshly laid but starts deteriorating progressively in relation to storage especially so under unfavourable environmental conditions. A fresh egg of high quality has a clean, sound and unbroken shell. The air cell located towards the large end is small and fixed in position. The white is composed of a large amount of thick albumen which is quite firm and viscous, even the thin white should not be too watery. The yolk is well centered and rises well above the surrounding thick albumen that is the yolk should have a good height, and a golden yellow colour. In addition to these, the egg should be free from any defects (blood spots, meat spots, etc.) which lowered consumer acceptance or render it inedible (germ development, rots, etc.).

Broadly, the following values may be regarded as representing the quality of fresh chicken eggs:

Egg character	Average value
Egg size, g.	55-58
Shape index	74-76
Air cell height,mm	2-3
Albumen Index	0.080-0.100
Yolk Index	0.55-0.45
Haugh Unit Score	80 and above
Shell thickness, mm	0.35-0.40

II. Deterioration during Storage

Egg starts deteriorating from the time it is laid. The first change which takes place in the egg after it is laid is loss of weight due to evaporation of moisture. Simultaneously there is also loss of carbon dioxide. The air cell at the blunt end of the egg begins to enlarge in the relation to the extent of evaporation. The thick albumen breaks down and becomes gradually more fluid and watery in character. The thin albumen increases in its content and spreads over a wide area, if examination on a flat surface after breaking the egg open.

There is transfer of water from the albumen to the yolk material through the vitelline membrane. The yolk becomes distended, flattened and tends to merge with the surrounding albumen. The penultimate stage of deterioration is reached when the thick white practically disappears, yolk becomes completely flattened and the vitelline membrane ruptures resulting in yolk and albumen getting mixed. The type of deteriorative changes is physio-chemical and microbiological in nature. In general, the extent of deteriorating that takes place will depend on storage temperature, humidity, length of storage and the degree of contamination. Among fertile eggs, spoilage due to embryonic development is an added factor.

III. Factors influencing egg quality

1. Genetic Influence or Breeding

High egg quality starts with breeding. A number of egg quality characteristics, such as egg size, shape, shell colour, shell thickness, albumen height, etc. are genetically controlled. Therefore, any programme aimed at improving egg quality must begin with a correct breeding policy. Even the incidence of blood and meat spots in the eggs has been shown to the under the influence of breeding. Hence, selection has to be exercised in order to keep such abnormal inclusions within tolerable limits.

2. Nutrition

A balanced diet is essential for production of eggs with high quality. The hen's diet can affect shell quality, colour of yolk, quality of albumen, incidence of blood spots and egg flavour. The content to Vitamin A, D and B complex. Vitamins (particularly riboflavin) of eggs is known to be dependent upon the amount of these vitamins in the feed. In order to produce eggs of good and uniform quality, adequate amounts of protein, vitamins, xanthophylls pigments and minerals, such as calcium and phosphorous, etc. are required and therefore, these nutrients should be regulated through proper dietary formulations to obtain desired results.

3. Management and Housing

Management and housing practices affect egg quality. Soiled or dietary eggs and cracked eggs can be kept at a minimum by avoiding overcrowding, keeping litter in good conditions, providing adequate number of nest holes and the use of sufficient and clean nesting material. In cage layer operations adequate slope and cushioning for the 'egg roll-out' requires attention to achieve good results and reduce breakages.

The fertility of eggs is another factor directly related to quality. Fertile eggs stored at room temperature soon become inedible, especially during summer months due to embryonic development. Therefore, only infertile eggs should be produced for table use and hatching eggs only for purposes of incubation. However, where fertile eggs are liable to enter the market for table purpose, it is better to defertilise such eggs soon after production so that they do not run the risk of germ development and consequential spoilage later on either in the market channels or in storage.

4. Diseases

Most outbreaks of disease or any major flock disturbances will influence egg quality. Notably Ranikhet Disease (RD) or New-castle Disease (ND) produces serious defects of both shell and egg contents. Infections Bronchitis also the similar effects. Layers affected by coryza, chronic respiratory disease, etc. are also likely to produce eggs of subnormal quality.

5. Age of Birds

Eggs laid by pullets during the first few months of production, though smaller in size are of the highest quality. This quality gradually tends to decline as the laying periods become extended. Egg shell quality also suffers with advancing age. However, the egg size becomes markedly better. Ever the season will affect egg quality being better in winter months and poor during the summer season.

6. Odours and Flavours

Eggs with off odours and fishy flavours have been reported when diets containing excessive amounts of fish meal, Cod-liver oil, certain waste materials, etc. are fed to layers. Eggs also readily absorb undesirable storage odours such as that of kerosene, onion, garlic and paints, etc. when stored in close proximity to such materials, thus lowering the acceptability of such eggs. It is quite desirable to pay proper attention to such aspects if highest consumer acceptance is to be obtained.

7. Microbial Contamination

Most freshly laid eggs are sterilising, at least inside i.e. egg contents. Surface contamination may occur from-faecal matter, nesting material or dirt. Contamination may also be contributed from handling and packaging materials. Micro organisms per shell, or hen's egg are reported to range from 10^2 to 10^7 with a mean of 10^5. The Types of micro organisms are diverse. In general, more spoilage is caused by bacteria than by moulds. Yeasts affect only occasionally. Even though bacterial and moulds are abundantly present on egg shell surface, contents seldom became contaminated because of eggs own defence mechanism to microbes. However, under certain conditions when microbes gain entry, the rich but highly perishable nutrients (human food) may readily undergo contamination and spoilage.

The micro-organisms encountered with eggs are mostly derived from he environment-air, water and soil, saprophytes or contaminates from faecal material. Plate counts greater than 10 million per ml (107) have been frequently associated with off odours, etc. while lower counts revealed no detectable or appreciable changes.

Some important or commonly found-organisms include the following genera:

a) Bacteria -Staphylococcis, Micrococci, Bacillus, Pseudomonas, Achromobacter, Proteus E. coli, etc.

b) Moulds or Fungi - Aspergillus, Pencillium, Alternaria and others.

c) Yeasts - Candidia, Trychosporon, Rhodotorula, etc.

8. Storage

Under storage conditions, temperature has been regarded as the most important single factor affecting egg quality. Both high temperature and low relative humidity adversely affect egg quality. At higher temperature there is increased weight loss due to evaporation and liquefective changes take place in the thick white. Also transfer t=of water from the albumen to the yolk causes the letter to become weak and flattened. These changes contribute to loss of quality directly proportional to the intensity of such changes. It should be appreciated that any measures which lowered the temperature, increase the humidity or curtail contamination will substantially aid in maintaining good quality during storage.

Egg Quality Determination

Egg quality denotes the characteristics of an egg which are preferred by the consumers. Determination or measurement of egg quality characteristics forms a pre-requisite for any improvement in egg quality, whether through methods of preservation or for consumer education and acceptance. Theoretically speaking, a variety of ways and methods have been evolved, developed and improved upon for better and more precise determination of egg quality. But from a practical stand point, the egg quality may be spoken only based upon the following two types :

i) Quality of egg that is broken open to study the contents ad constituents more precisely.

ii) Quality of the intact egg (shell egg) by candling.

The former furnishes a deeper insight into egg quality and is largely used for purposes of research findings, breeding programmes and in relation to advance the cause of poultry technology. The latter has been specially developed for measuring quality of market eggs i.e. shell eggs.

Regardless of the objectives some common measures of egg quality are based on size, shape, cleanliness and shell quality (External quality measurements) and such factors like albumen height, diameter of thick and thin albumen, albumen index,-yolk height, diameter of thick and thin albumen, yolk colour, etc. Internal quality measurements and the candled appearance foe shell eggs (Market quality measurement). The various quality attributes mentioned above have been dealt with in detail elsewhere in this manual appropriately under Theory or Laboratory Exercises which may please be referred to for fuller in format on.

Care and Handling of Eggs on the Farm

It is important to produce and market egg of high quality with an attractive appearance and to adopt measures to reduce the risk of their spoilage. Naturally clean eggs (nest-clean) are more attractive and save labour and money that is involved in processing dirty eggs. It is equally important to produce infertile eggs for table purpose so that there is no danger of spoilage from embryonic or germ development. In modern times, it is almost become universal practice to produce clean and infertile eggs in a routine way. Producing good quality eggs is an integral part of organised farming activity. Careful adoption of simple but important practices on the farm can go a long way in producing eggs of high quality. The following practices are recommended :

1. Confinement of Laying Flocks

Complete confinement system whether on litter or in cages makes it easy to produce infertile eggs. Better control over the rations is possible and more uniform egg quality, yolk colour, and shell quality can be obtained.

2. Dry Litter Floor

The litter should be kept reasonably clean and dry eggs enhancing the scope of microbiological contamination and spoilage. Not only the litter, even the nesting material should be clean and renewal periodically to maintain sufficient quality to assist the production of clean eggs and reduces the chances of breakages.

3. Frequent Gathering of Eggs

Loss of egg quality may occur during the time interval between laying and gathering of eggs. Hence, frequent gathering of eggs from layer houses is desirable especially from litter houses. Eggs should be gathered three to four times a day depending -upon the number of layers, density conditions, nesting space available, rate of production and labour involved, etc. Even under cage operations eggs are usually gathered about twice a day.

4. Collection of Eggs in Wire baskets or Filler Flats:

It is better to collect eggs in suitable type of wire baskets or filler flats because this permits better circulation of air between the eggs than when closed containers, such as buckets, boxes, etc. are used. Collection of eggs directly into filler flats will further reduce handling and breakages.

5. Handling and Packing Eggs Properly

It is important to pack all eggs with the large end upper most and to see that rough handling is avoided. It is also necessary to quickly cool eggs conserve quality.

6. Eggs should be Stored Properly

Proper attention to storage of eggs is an essential requirement. Both the conditions and length of storage exert a pronounced influence on egg quality. In this connection a general principle to remember is that a low temperature and high humidity preserve egg quality. However, for ideal storage of eggs, some kind of refrigerated facilities become almost a necessity, depending upon the duration of storage, the quantum of eggs stored, etc.

7. Preservation Methods are Helpful

Several methods of egg preservation are available. The choice of method to be adopted will be governed by such conditions as, cost, available, facilities, case of application, quantity of eggs being handled, labour require and the duration of storage. Any convenient method may be adopted. As a general rule, some method of preservation is better that no preservation at all, especially so in relation to the length of time from production to consumption and the environmental temperatures, season of the year, etc.

8. Eggs should be Marketed Frequently

Eggs should be marketed at least twice a week and more often in summer months. Frequency of marketing will be conditioned by the size of the flock, processing and preservation done and method of shipment. It is important to move eggs rapidly through marketing channels, if the eggs reach the consumers with good quality.

Handling and Cleaning of Dirty Eggs

In the first instance efforts must be directed towards production of clean eggs. However, it is well known that some dirty eggs (5-10%) are inevitably seen on the farm, more so on litter floors. Such eggs which are dirty should be handled separately using any one of the two procedures : i) Cleaning ii) Washing.

1. Cleaning of Dirty Eggs

The eggs may be dry-cleaned by hand, only if slightly stained. For this purpose a fine emery cloth or sand paper mounted on a wooden frame is used for buffing the eggs. This process removes visible dirt but is slow and does not clean badly soiled eggs and can be associated with breakage.

2. Washing of Dirty Eggs

In instances where large quantity of dirty eggs are to be handled (e.g. Large size farms, marketing centres, wholesalers, etc.), it is desirable to wash the eggs. Egg washing must be practices only where proper facilities exist for the purpose. For proper washing of eggs, an egg washing machine, a suitable detergent-sanitizer and correct procedure should be employed to achieve satisfactory results. As a matter of normal practice, only non-odourous, non-toxic detergent-sanitizers (hypochlorite or other compounds, etc.) at the rate of 20-25 grams per bucket of water (15-16 litres) maintained at a temperature of 43-48^{0}C (110-120^{0}F) are used for machine washing for about 2-3 minutes. Fresh solution is used and renewed after washing 500-600 eggs.

3. General precautions

As a matter of general precaution, it is very important to remember the following while dealing with dirty eggs :

1. Only excessively soiled and dirty eggs should be washed.
2. Cracked and thin shelled eggs are not washed because of breakages involved.
3. Dirty eggs should be washed as soon as possible.
4. Eggs should never be washed with plain water. Only recommended detergent-sanitizer should be used.

5. Washed eggs should not be stored but marketed as early as possible.
6. Washed eggs should be marketed separately preferably within a week because of their poor shelf life.

Candling and Grading of Eggs

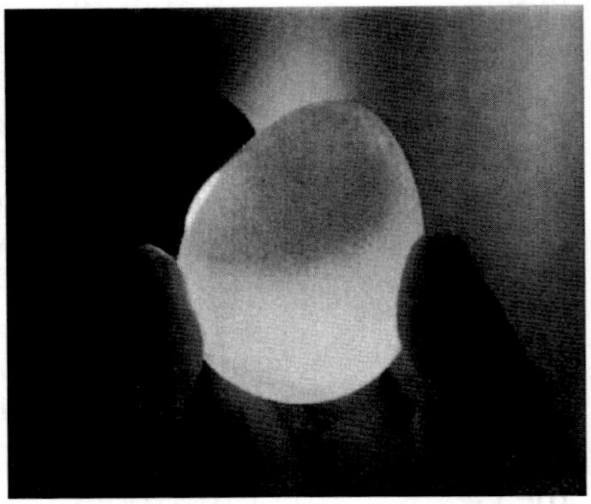

The commercial practice for evaluating the quality of shell eggs is by candling. This method consists of holding the egg before a suitable light (candling light) and looking at the illuminated shell to determine the condition, of its contents. The measures of quality are based on the appearance of shell, air cell, yolk and albumen.

The term, "Grading" generally refers to sorting of products according to quality, size, weight and other factors that determine the relative value of the product. The grading of shell eggs is the classifying of individual egg according to the established standards. In the grading of eggs, they are classified according to their weight, (that is the size) either expressed in grams per egg or ounces per dozen eggs.

In effect, candling and grading of eggs is done with a view to enable grouping of eggs into lots having similar characteristics of quality and weight.

Facilities for Candling and Grading

Certain facilities are required for proper candling and grading of eggs. These requirements may be considered as follows:

1. Candling Room
2. Candling Bench
3. Candling Light
4. Weighing/Grading Equipment

1. Candling Room

This facility is necessary for large scale candling and grading work. The candling room should be darkened to the extent necessary to facilitate an efficient job. There should be no cross beams of light between the person candling the eggs and the candling light, except those emanating from the egg Candler. The candling light aperture should be no placed that rays of light coming from it will not shine directly into the graders eyes when he is in position for candling.

It is desirable that the walls and coiling of the candling room have smooth washable surfaces which are painted with a dark coloured, flat-finish paint to avoid light, reflection. The linear work space provided for each person will depend largely on the number of eggs and grades being handled.

The floors should be strong, washable and provided with drains. Adequacy of water supply for cleaning the room is another requirement. Sufficient overhead lights should be provided to help in the cleaning up of the room.

For small-scale candling and grading work, even an appropriate "Candling Booth" of sufficient size, darkefied properly by black curtains and provided with suitable facilities should also serve the purpose well.

2. Candling Bench

The candling bench or grading bench or the work table of a suitable height (0.8 to 1 mtr) is required so that eggs can be viewed comfortably against the candling light. While the size and design, etc. may vary according to actual needs, it must be remembered that sufficient shelf space is available for stacking eggs, egg trays, cartons and cases, etc. space should also be availble for dealing with eggs which do not qualify for being marketed or those condemned and rejected.

In some large-scale modern operations, more elaborate and automatic facilities are usually used; fitted with specialized equipment and a particular room lay-out.

3. Candling Light

There are many styles and types of candling lights that have been commercially used, with varying light intensity and size of the aperture. Regardless of the type, candling light (also called lamp, egg Candler, etc.) should provide comfort and proper illumination.

The candling light usually consists of an electric bulb enclosed in a metal or wooden box or container or reflector-type housing with an aperture of about 2.5 to 3.0 cms. in diameter and often a cushioned ring. The beam of light (which is brighter when reflectors are used) merges from the aperture and passé through the egg which is held against it, thus illuminating the egg contents better. The candling light is so adjusted in height that the person viewing the eggs. A candling light delivering 350-450 foot-candles of light is desirable, for which purpose a 60-75 watt bulb is sufficient.

4. Weighing Equipment

The candling bench or the candling room should be equipped with proper egg scales. In commercial plants, every egg is not weighed, rather the sight and tough is used for determining weight of eggs which may be verified using a scale if doubt arises. Many automatic and semi-automatic devices have been developed and installed for "On-the-line egg grading operations". Even equipments which combine candling and weighing procedures have become very popular in bulk-handling of eggs in large modern commercial units in advanced countries.

Candled Appearance of Eggs

The egg is placed at the candling aperture with the air cell upwards and titled slightly away from the observer and by twirling or rotating the egg, the shell and contents are viewed. Eggs of good or high quality show clean, sound and unbroken shells. The air cell located towards the large and (broad end) is small and fixed.

The egg contents appear pinkish yellow, the yolk casting a dim or indistinct shadow and float close to the centre but rotate freely as the egg is twirled. Moving along with the yolk, often a faint spot can also be seen. This is the chalaza, Good quality eggs have clear and firm albumen which is so thick that the yolk does not move freely.

Eggs which show signs of germ development or such defects as blood spots, meat spots or rots, etc. are rendered inedible or unfit for human consumption. Since quality is based on human judgement, sufficient practice and experience is required to obtain accuracy and speed.

Certain terms, etc. are generally used while assessing the candled quality of eggs. Common or important terms used and their description are given. Read these carefully and understand the various terminologies that are applicable.

Advantages of Grading

Although classifying eggs according to quality and weight involves time, labour and money, it has its own advantages under a well-organised poultry farming activity and improved marketing methods. The necessity for egg grading will however depend largely upon the choice of consumers. Some important advantages of grading are given below:

1. The producer and consumers will be compelled to evince greater interest and quality awareness, with better satisfaction to the consumer.
2. Grading reduces confusion or uncertainty in respect of egg quality.
3. It provides a uniform standard for measuring differences in quality.
4. It enables pooling of eggs of comparable quality coming from different sources.
5. It provides a basis for settlement of disputes involving quality between producers, sellers and consumers.
6. Market prices reports for various grades are more easily understood.
7. Standards can provide a basis for advertising and sales promotion.
8. They expand consumer demand by making possible lower grades at lower prices and superior grades for higher prices. The Indian Standards for grading of eggs are tabulated.

Table 3: Grade designation and detailed specifications according to Indian Standards (ISI) for the quality of shell eggs

Grade	Weight per egg (g)	Shell	Air cell	White	Yolk
A-Extra large A-Large A-Medium A-Small	60 and above 53-59 45-52 38-44	Clean, unbroken and sound Shape normal	Upto 4 mm in depth practically regular or better	Clear, reasonably firm	Fairly well centred, practically free from defects. Outline indistinct.
B-Extra large B-Large B-Medium B-Small	60 and above 53-59 45-52 36-44	Clean to moderately stained and sound, shape slightly abnormal	8 mm or less in depth, may be free and slightly bubbly	Clear may be slightly weak	May be slightly off centred. Outline slightly visible

Note

i) Eggs not conforming to the above grades may be debarred from entering trade channels as fresh shell eggs.

iii) Two grades 'A' and 'B' and four size/weight classifications are provided under these grades.

Terms Descriptive of the Shell

Clean

A shell that is free from foreign material and form stains or discolorations that are readily visible. An egg may be considered clean if it has only very small speck of stains, if such specks or stains are not of sufficient number of intensity to detract from the generally clean appearance of the egg. Eggs that show traces of processing oil on the shell are considered clean unless otherwise soiled.

Dirty

A shell has dirt adhering to its surface or which has prominent stains or slight to moderate stains covering more that of the shell surface.

Checked or Cracked

A shell that has an actual break or broach but its membranes are unbroken and its contents do not leak.

Body check

A body check is an egg in which the shell appears to have been cracked while in the uterus presumably before all of the shell material was formed. The break is then sealed by the deposition of additional shell material, so tht after being laid it appears normal at causal inspection. The work shell is detected only by candling.

Leaker

An egg, the shell and membranes of which are broken to the extent that the egg contents are leaking or free to lack through the shell.

Abnormal

A shell that may be decidedly misshapen or faulty in texture or strength or may show pronounced fridges, thin spots or rough areas.

Terms Descriptive of the Air Cell

Depth of air cell

The depth of the air cell is the distance from its top to its bottom when the egg is held air cell upward, it can be measured using an air cell gauge.

Practically regular

An air cell that maintains a practically fixed position in the egg and shows fairly even outline, with not more than inch movement in any direction as the egg is rotated.

Free Air cell

An air cell that move freely towards the upper most point in the egg as the egg is rotated slowly.

A ruptured air cell resulting in one or more small separate air bubbles usually floating beneath main air cell.

Terms Descriptive of the White

Clear

A white that is free from any discoloration or from any foreign bodies in it. (Prominent chalazae should not be confused with foreign bodies, such as spots or blood clots).

Firm

A white that is sufficiently thick or viscous to permit only limited movement of the yolk from the centre of the egg, thus preventing the yolk outline from being more than slightly defined or indistinctly indicated, when the egg is twirled.

Weak and Watery

A white that is thin and generally lacking in viscosity. A weak and watery white permits the yolk to move freely from the centre of the egg and to approach the shell closely, thus causing the yolk outline to appear plainly visible and dark when the egg is twirled.

Blood clots and Spots: (Not due to germ development) react

Blood clots or spots on the surface of the yolk or floating in the white. These blood clots may have lot their red colour and appear as meat spots. If they are not over 1/8 inch in diameter, the egg may be allowed. If larger or showing diffusion of blood in the white surrounding them, the egg will be classified as loss.

Terms Descriptive of Yolk

Well Centred

A yolk that occupies the centre of the egg and moves only slightly fro that position as the egg is twirled.

Off Centre

A yolk is distinctly above or below centre and swings close to the sides of the egg as it is twirled.

Outline Slightly Defined

A yolk outline that is indistinctly indicated and appears to blend into the surrounding white as the egg is twirled.

Enlarges and Flattened

A yolk in which the yolk membranes and tissues have weakened and moisture has been absorbed from the white to such an extent that it appears definitely enlarges and flat.

Free from Defects

A yolk that shows no spots or areas on its surface indicating the presence of germ development or other.

Serious Defects

A yolk shows well developed spots or areas and other serious defects, such as olive yolks, which do not render the egg inedible.

Clearly Visible Germ Development

A development of the germ spot on the yolk of a fertile egg that has progressed to appoint where it is plainly visible as definite circular area or spot with no blood in evidence.

Blood due to Germ Development

Blood caused by development of the germ in a fertile egg to the point where it is visible as definite lines or as a blood ring. Such an egg is classed inedible.

General Terms

Loss

An egg that is inedible, smashed or broken so that the contents are leaking, contaminated or containing bloody whites, large blood or meat spots or other foreign material.

Inedible Eggs

Eggs of the following description are classed as inedible. Black rots, white rots, mixed rots (addled eggs), sour eggs, eggs with green whites, eggs with stuck yolks, mouldy eggs, musty eggs, egg showing blood rings, eggs containing embryo, chicks, and eggs that have absorbed offensive odours.

Preservation and Storage of Shell Eggs

Preservation of eggs can be considered under two groups:

i) Preservation of shell eggs

ii) Preservation of liquid processed eggs (after breaking open)

Under this topic, only preservation and storage of shell eggs will be dealt with. It is important to remember that egg quality is the sum total of all the characteristics that influence the acceptability by consumers. Shell eggs are prone to deteriorate or spoil in the market channels or in storage due to a variety of causes. Lowered quality or spoilage in shell eggs may be brought about by such factors as: embryonic development, shrinkage of contents, breakdown of albumen and water transfer (liquefaction), microbiological contamination, etc.

Therefore it is essential that shell eggs are properly and adequately preserved so that their quality does not suffer adversely in market channels. The various methods of preservation may b classified in different ways. Some are well suited to village conditions, others for farm level usage, whereas some are only of commercial importance. Briefly, these are listed below:

1. Immersion Methods (water glass and lime reeling method)
2. Oil treatment (Oil dipping and spraying)
3. Heat treatment (Thermo-stabilization)
4. Refrigerated storage (Short-term and Long-term storage).

The requirements and importance of these methods is dealt with. It is worthy of emphasis that any preservation method does not improve the quality of poor eggs and hence only good quality eggs can benefit from preservation methods by retarding decline in quality.

1. Immersion Methods

This method of preserving shell eggs is a fairly old but satisfactory procedure for retaining egg quality in village conditions or on small farms or elsewhere involving preservation of smaller lots of infertile eggs. Immersion methods require only simple techniques and much equipments, nut the following prerequisites :

a) Only infertile, fresh and good quality eggs should be used.

b) Materials used for preservation should not impart any undesirable taste or odour.

c) Prepared solutions should not deteriorate even under long periods of storage.

d) Should prevent gaseous exchange between eggs and the atmosphere.

e) It should satisfactorily protect the edible quality of eggs under storage.

Water Glass Method

It is one of the old, household methods regarded as satisfactory or treating a few dozen eggs. For this purpose water (previously boiled and cooled) is poured into a clean jar or container (Plastic, earthen, cemented or wooden) and water glass (sodium silicate) is added to make an approximately 10% solution. After thoroughly mixing the solution fresh, clean and infertile eggs are gently lowered into the cooled water glass solution and kept completely immersed. The eggs can then be withdrawn and stored at room temperature. The colloids adsorb and block the shell pores without any chemical reaction, thus preserving egg quality.

Lime Sealing Method

Limewater can be used equally satisfactorily for preserving the eggs. Limewater is prepared by mixing one part of quicklime (Calcium Oxide, CaO) with about four to five parts of water solution. The mixture is stirred well and allowed to stand overnight and the clear liquid on decanting can be used for immersion of eggs. The jar container which should be non-corrosive is covered and kept in a cool place. It is beneficial to add a sufficient quantity of salt (approximately ½ to 1 part with a view to increase the specific gravity of the solution so that eggs do not strike the bottom of the container and get broken, when immersed. Maximum advantage is obtained after the eggs are left dipped in limewater for 14 to 16 hrs. This results in the shells becoming coated with calcium carbonate. Eggs could then be removed and stored at room temperature.

Immersion method is for egg preservation give satisfactory protection to egg quality. Such eggs keep well under room temperature for about 2 to 3 weeks depending upon the environment. It is important to use only eggs with good shell quality, otherwise they would be prone to crack and breakages.

2. Oil Treatment

Eggs may be oil treated using suitable, light weight, mineral oils which are colourless, odourless and tasteless, e.g., Liquid paraffin, etc. however, commercial egg-coating oils have been evolved and are availble that have given better results. The oil may be used for spraying (oil spraying) using a hand or electric sprayer or for immersing the eggs.

Oil Spraying

The eggs are held in egg filler floss with the broad end up and oil sprayed to cover half to three-fourth of the shell surface. This accomplishes spraying which satisfactorily preserved egg quality for two to three weeks. About 400 ml. of oil is sufficient for treating 1000 eggs.

Oil Dipping

In this method, eggs are dipped in mineral oil until completely immersed (oil dipping) and withdrawn an allowed to stand to drain off the excess oil. This oil could be heated, filtered, cooled and reused. Oil dipped eggs are preserved instantaneously and give better protection to egg quality is pre-warmed to maintain the temperature slightly higher than that of eggs required to be dipped. Approximately 400 ml. of oil is required for 200 to 250 eggs. This makes it relatively expensive and also involves more labour than the oil-spraying method but has given superior results in quality retention.

Advantages of Oil Treatment

1. Reduces the escape of carbondioxide and moisture from the egg by blocking the shell pores.
2. Keeps out bacteria and odours (egg coating oils often contain bactericides and fungicides).
3. Prevents weightloss
4. Maintains good internal quality
5. Where suitable oil is available, the procedure is simple.

3. Heat Treatment

The stabilisation of egg quality by the use of heat treatment method is called thermo-stabilisation. Of special significance is its suitability in preserving the quality of even fertile eggs (fresh) by destroying the viable germ (blastoderm). For this purpose, water which is heated and maintained at a definite temperature is used for placing eggs, and stirring, using specific time for heat treatment.

Several combinations of temperature and duration have been tried to affect a hundred per cent kill of the blastoderm and to obtain maximum quality stabilisation. Usually eggs are thermo-stabilised by immersing shell eggs for 15 to 20 minutes at 55 degree Celsius, while the water is kept stirred although. This results in a fine film of peripheral albumen immediately next to the shell becoming coagulated. Proper control of time and temperature is necessary to achieve satisfactory results without cooking the contents.

Advantages of Thermo-stabilisation

1. It is the method of choice in the preservation of fertile eggs (but before any appreciable embryonic growth). Hence, it forms an effective procedure for dealing with eggs produced in villages, etc. because it defertilises the eggs.
2. Kills bacteria on the egg shell surface extending storage life.
3. The fine layer of cooked albumen retards physic-chemical changes in egg contents. Thereby, improving the keeping quality of eggs.
4. Permits room temperature storage of thermo-stabilised eggs for 3 to 4 weeks, depending upon the environmental conditions.

4. Refrigerated Storage

Eggs intended for cold storage must be carefully candled to remove dirty, cracked and low quality eggs. The eggs are then held at a temperature of 0 degree Celsius (30-32 degree F) and a relative humidity of about 90%. Under such refrigerated conditions of storage, eggs can be preserved for 5-8 months. For short term preservation (3-4 wks), eggs can be stored at a temperature of 10-20 degree C (50-55 degree F) with a relative humidity of 60-70%. It should be borne in mind that egg freezes at 28 degree F or minus 2 degree C hence, cold storage temperature should definitely be higher than this. It may also be noted that cold storage conditions do not allow any embryonic growth.

Refrigerated storage required a suitable room (well-insulated), free from abnormal odours and flavours, as well as the availability of electricity and refrigerated facilities. Though, undoubtedly the best method, cold storage is a very costly procedure.

5. Combination of Methods

Sometimes a combination of any two compatible methods has been preferred to a single one. Such procedures are doubt more cumbersome and costly and have been used only to a limited extend to prolong the shelf life of eggs, e.g., oil treatment with cold storage, thermo-stabilization and oil-coating (i.e. simultaneous thermo-stabilization and oil treatment by thermo-stabilization in oil).

❑❑❑

Chapter **4**

Incubation & Hatching

The hatchery business has become a specialised branch of Poultry industry due to its rapid development in recent years. Now-a-days very a large number of hatcheries have been established all over India. Poultry farmers obtain their requirements of chicks from commercial hatcheries.

Hatching

Hatching is the production of baby chicks from fertile eggs. In early days, eggs were hatched by placing them under broody hens and desi hens were ideal for this purpose. The normal incubation period of chicken eggs is 21 days, although there is some variation in each direction. The eggs of Leghorn and other light breeds commonly hatch a few hours earlier than those of the heavier breeds.

Methods of Incubation

There are two methods of incubation usually practical as:

a) Natural Incubation

b) Artificial Incubation

a) Natural Incubation

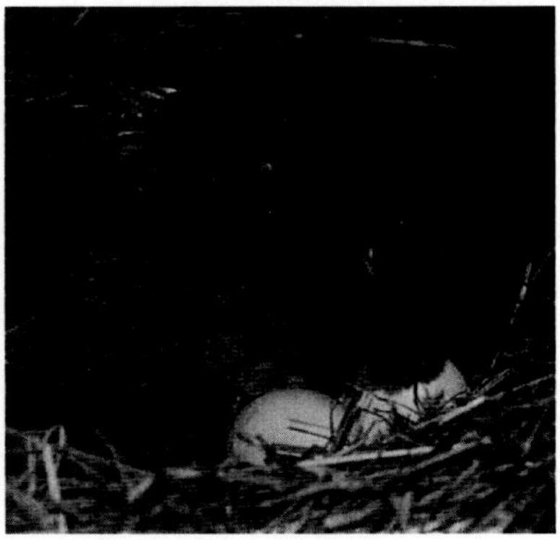

Natural Incubation of eggs

This method is popular with small poultry keepers in remote rural area of the country. Broodiness, the desire to hatch out chicks out of fertile eggs is a natural instinct in female birds. This behaviour is made use of during natural incubation. Although this method is fast disappearing and being replaced by artificial method. It is worthwhile to consider different aspects of natural method of incubation. A broody hen used for incubating eggs should be healthy, quite a good sitter and should have a good body size. She may be tested with help dummy eggs for her interest to sit on eggs. She should be tested for internal and external parasites before allowing her to sit on eggs.

A saucer-shaped nest made of bamboo basket or wooden box filled with bedding material should be provided at safe and comfortable place. Depending upon the size of the hen, 10-15 eggs can be placed under one hen. The hen should be taken out at least twice a day for about 30 minutes to be fed and watered. During hot summer, it may be necessary to sprinkle the eggs with small quantity of water to maintain the humidity. The hen takes care of newly hatched chicks.

b) Artificial Incubation

Artificial method of incubation of eggs is known to man for more than 2000 years and the earliest record of incubation are from China and Egypt. The early Chinese appear to have utilised the heat of sotting manure for hatching eggs. Later they used charcoal fire in cylindrical oven made of earthen materials with a combined smoke hole and variable damper at the base for incubating eggs. The egg baskets held in the overseen to have several layers of eggs. The ancient Egyptian used artificial incubation on large scale. Their incubators were built of mud bricks and consisted of central corridor. On either side of the corridor was a series of ovens of standard pattern. The egg chambers were at ground level and had ground level and had opening in corridor for attending the chicks and eggs in the chambers. Above the egg chambers were the heating compartments.

Types of Incubators

Commercial incubators are of two principal designs, the sectional or still-air type and the cabinet or forced draft type. The mammoth type incubator are essentially the cabinet type, the only difference being in the capacity of that can be hatched.

There are large room type incubators called walk-incubators with a capacity of hold thousands of eggs at a time.

1. Sectional type or still air type

The sectional type incubator is usually of small capacity ranging from 50-500 eggs, with single layer incubation. Depending on the air movement, they are known as still air type because there is practically no air movement in this type of incubators. In such units, heat is generally transmitted by conduction inside the egg chamber either through hot water tanks or hot air tubes. The temperature is controlled by a thermostat and humidity is maintained by water pans kept inside the incubator. Ventilation is provided through port holes (air vents) which consists of air inlets and exhaust.

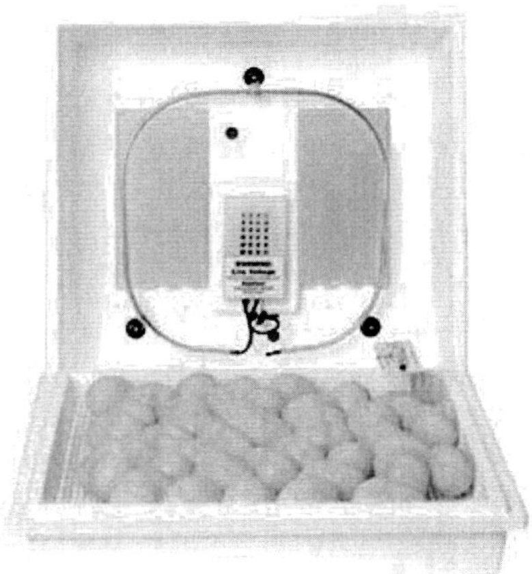

Sectional type or still air type incubator

2. The cabinet type or Forced draft type or Mammoth type

The cabinet type incubators are an improvement on the sectional type machines as to the capacity of eggs that can be incubated in a smaller space because of super imposing of many layers of eggs. They are known as forced draft type because the air is evenly distributed with the help of mechanical draft (by a fan) inside the egg cabinet. The arrangements for temperature control, humidity and ventilation are by thermostat, humidistat and air inlet and exhaust respectively. The turning of eggs is either mechanical or automatically carried out (motorised). The arrangement of setter and Hatcher trays could be made in the same machine or in different machines as per the model of the manufacturers. Incubators are generally operated by electricity. On the basis of heat transmission system used, they can further be considered either as hot water or hot air type. The hot water machines are still air and sectional type as the heat is transmitted by conduction which cannot be efficiently utilised for large incubators. The hot air type machines are commonly the forced draft type incubators, wherein, the air inside the egg chamber is heated and uniformly distributed.

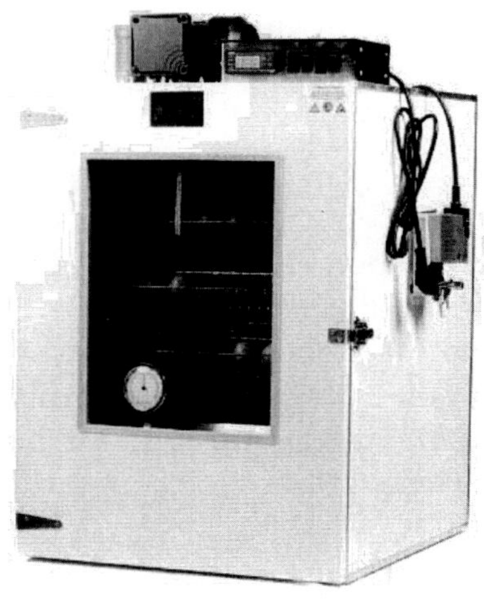

Cabinet type incubator

Physical Requisites for Incubation

Whether the process of incubation is carried out in natural way under a broody hen or in a mechanical incubator, certain physical criteria in respect of temperature, humidity, turning and ventilation have to be maintained. These conditions are created in natural incubation, by broody hens but under artificial incubation, an incubator has to be operated well to maintain the above conditions. The following requirements should be fully controlled and maintained. It is important to follow the recommendations of the manufacturers of incubators to obtain best hatching results.

a) Temperature

Control of temperature is the most critical single factor for the successful hatching of eggs. Developing embryos are extremely sensitive to temperature of the environment.

Slight variation in temperature may mean the difference between high and low hatchability. Temperature has an effect not only on hatchability but also on quality of hatch. It has direct effect on time taken for hatching, embryo size, embryo mortality and viability of chicks produced.

Species of birds vary in their temperature requirement for incubation. In forced draft incubators used for incubating eggs of poultry species temperature varies from 37.2 to 37.7°C depending upon their construction. In setter-cum-Hatcher, the same temperature is maintained throughout the incubation period and where the Hatcher is separate temperature is slightly reduced to 35.5 to 36.5°C in hatchers.

Effect of high temperature depends upon the degree of increase in temperature above optimum and the length of time, the high temperature is maintained. It results in high embryonic mortality particularly when there is high temperature during the last part of incubation period (19th day onward in case of chicken eggs). High temperature during early stages of incubation was not followed by immediate mortality of embryos but death was delayed until near hatching time. Other effects of high incubation temperature are smaller chicks, lack of alertness in chicks, crooked toes, spraddled legs, crooked neck, etc. high incubation temperature shortness the incubation time by several hours. But exposure of eggs to 46°C for 3 hours or 49°C for one hour kills all embryos. The thermostat controlling the temperature should be checked regularly with thermometers of known accuracy used. The actual temperature should be checked when the pilot light goes off, that is when the thermostat control cuts off the heat. The temperature is Hatcher should be heat generated by embryonated eggs themselves raise the temperature beyond critical level.

The incubation temperature below the normal caused late hatch and poor hatchability.

b) Humidity

Proper level of humidity in the incubator is an important as temperature for obtaining good hatches. In the mammoth incubators, automatic control of humidity is maintained by filling moisture trays with water and also by controlling the air vents. The optimum humidity is 60% which is indicated by a wet bulb reading of 36.6 degree with a dry bulb temperature of 38°C. During hatching period, the humidity is increased to give a wet bulb reading of 32-33°C.

Slight errors in maintaining humidity in either setters or the hatchers will not be as determined as fluctuate in temperature. Low humidity during incubation results in excessive water loss from the eggs. The effect will be small, hard chicks. If the humidity is too low in hatchers, there will be incidence of piped eggs and embryos are dried out in the shell or dead in the shell.

High humidity during incubation prevents sufficient evaporation from the eggs resulting in large soggy chicks. High humidity also has a tendency to delay hatch and reduce hatchability. The chicks will have poorly headed navels. Shell will be sticking to chicks.

c) Ventilation

Embryos use oxygen for their metabolism and give off carbon dioxide. The concentration of these gases in the air has a significant effect on hatchability. Air contains 21% oxygen and this seems to be the optimum concentration for the developing embryo. Any fall in oxygen below this level results in a lowered percentage of hatch. For every per cent reduction in oxygen content, there is decrease of 5% hatchability and for every percent increase beyond 21 per cent hatchability decreases by one per cent.

The carbon dioxide concentration in incubator should range between 0.3 to 0.5 per cent for maximum hatchability. Concentration above 1 per cent increases embryonic mortality and at 5 per cent concentration of carbon dioxide for prolonged period all the embryos die. The internal fan speed or RPM should be roughly 7200 rpm.

d) Turning of Eggs

The eggs should be turned gently by the mechanical device provided in the setter to prevent their settling and adhering to other structures of eggs. In still-air type of incubators turning of eggs also insures the even heating of the egg contacts. Modern incubators are equipped with turning devices that are able to rotate egg trays through an angle of 90 degrees. These are controlled by a timing mechanism and usually eggs are turned every hour. At least 6-8 turning a day at regular intervals are needed for better hatchability. No turning is required for chicken eggs after the 18th day of incubation.

e) Position of egg in the incubator

Eggs are normally incubated large end up-under these conditions, the head of the embryo develop at the large end of the egg near the air cell. When eggs are incubated small end up the majority of embryos develop with their heads in the small end of the egg and frequently these embryos do not hatch.

Table 1: Incubation requirements for various species of poultry

Species	Incubation Period (days)	Temperature (F)	Humidity (%)	Do not turn after	Humidity for last 3 days (%)
Chicken	21	100	85-87	18th day	90
Turkey	28	99	84-86	25th day	90
Duck	28	100	85-86	25th day	90
Muscovy duck	35-37	100	85-86	31th day	90
Goose	28-34	99	86-88	25th day	90
Guinea fowl	28	100	85-87	25th day	90
Pheasant	23-28	100	86-88	21th day	92
Pea fowl	28-30	99	84-86	2th day	90
Bob white quail	28-24	100	84-87	20th day	90
Coturnix quail	17	100	85-86	15th day	90
Pigeon	17	100	85-87	15th day	90

Selection of Hatching Eggs

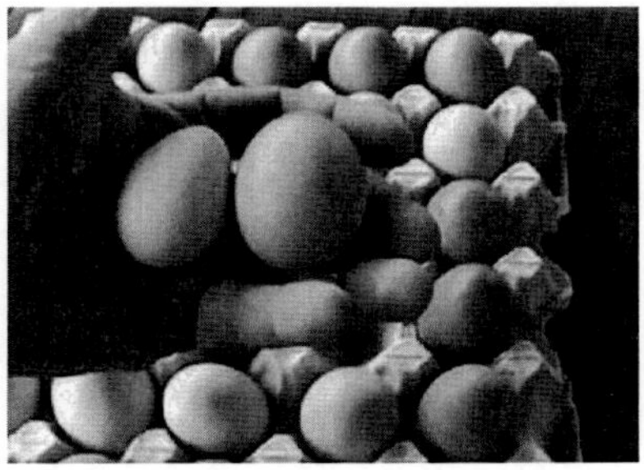

The successful production of high quality chicks begins with the breeder. Chicks that will be used for the production of eggs or poultry meat should be derived from breeding flocks selected on the basis of desired characteristics of egg or meat production. Breeders should be disease-free, fed an adequate diet and maintained under conditions that are conductive to successful mating. Unfortunately there is no way of telling, if an egg is fertile ot not prior to incubation, without opening it. Thus, if fertility is not high, many eggs will be set that do not develop embryos and many eggs are wasted because the infertile-incubated eggs are not remarkable.

Hatching eggs should be selected with care because certain abnormalities adversely affect hatchability. Therefore, eggs that have characteristics associated with poor hatchability should be discarded. Some important characters for selection of hatching eggs are size, shape, shell quality and interior quality as observed by candling.

1. Size of eggs

The egg size is related to hatchability. Extremely large and small eggs do not hatch well. Therefore, medium-sized eggs should be selected for hatching (50-55g). The proportion of thick white is high in a very large egg and low in very small ones which interfere with normal hatchability.

2. Shape of eggs

The shape of hatching eggs should be ovoid. Eggs of abnormal shape do not hatch well. However, eggs that are only slightly off shape, ridged or wrinkled generally hatch as good as normal shaped eggs, though they are more prone to breakage during incubation. Therefore, preference is for eggs of normal shape.

3. Shell Quality

Eggs with sound shell should be selected. The quality of shell is related to hatchability because the shell serves as a protective cover, provides a means of gaseous exchange and supplies necessary calcium for the developing embryo. Some strains and family of layers produce weak shells. The shell thickness declines during hot weather also. Further, calcium nutrition of the bird will also affect the shell thickness. Thin shelled eggs do not generally hatch well due to increased evaporative loss during incubation. Besides, there are more losses due to breakage of eggs having thin and weak shells. Therefore, care must be exercised in the selection of eggs for hatching and only those with strong and normal shells should be selected.

Clean eggs hatch better than the soiled eggs because soiling substances seal the pores of the shell, interfering with air movement through the shell to the embryo. Dirt also harbours micro-organisms rendering eggs more prone to spoilage. Slightly soiled eggs could be dry cleaned and used for hatching while excessively soiled ones are not suitable.

4. Interior quality

On candling egg that show inferior market quality, such as loose air cells, blood spots, meat spots, hair cracks and poor interior quality do not hatch well. Therefore, eggs with good interior quality, showing an indistinct yolk shadow, small air cell and good albumen condition upon candling should be chosen for hatching to obtain good results.

Care of Hatching Eggs

It is important to handle hatching eggs properly and carefully before incubation to achieve maximum hatchability of viable and strong chicks. The following care may be necessary:

1. Collection of egg

Gather the hatching eggs as frequently as possible, particularly in severe weathers. Three or four gatherings of eggs from poultry shed will be necessary to avoid undue effect of weather on embryos.

2. Storage temperature

It is important that eggs should be stored below "Physiological zero" temperature or temperature at which there is almost no embryonic development which is approximately 21.1°C without adversely affecting the hatching power of the eggs. But beyond this range hatchability is affected adversely depending upon the duration of storage. Hatchability starts declining rapidly, when eggs are stored at 0°C. In the same way when eggs are stored at 32.2°C for 7 days, embryos are completely destroyed. Pre-warming is beneficial, if eggs are stored at 10%C. A pre-warming temperature of 23°C for 18 hours before setting eggs in incubator is recommended.

3. Humidity

High humidity is preferred over the low humidity, particularly when the storage temperature is high to abide drying of the eggs. A relative humidity of 80% during storage appears to be the nest. If eggs are to be stored for 2 to 3 weeks, they may be sealed in gas impermeable pack and flushed with nitrogen gas.

4. Handling of egg

Hatching egg should be stored in hard, clean filler flats keeping small end down. Eggs held with their large end down and eggs handled roughly develop tremulous air cells. Such eggs with loose air cells do not hatch well. Rough handling may result in cracked eggs as well which seldom hatch.

Ordinarily, hatching eggs may not be held for more than a week but if they are required to be held longer, they should be turned at regular intervals, right from the first day, to improve the hatchability. The turning of eggs, during holding periods, longer than one week prevents the blastoderm from sticking to the shell.

5. Age of eggs or length of storage

The length of time eggs can be held without lowering hatchability depends on the temperature at which eggs are held. Generally, eggs held at 10-15°C can be stored for one week, thereafter, hatchability declines progressively. In eggs held upto 4 weeks hatchability is almost completely lost. Therefore, hatching eggs should be set at least once a week, while twice is preferable.

6. Cleanliness of the shell

As a general rule, only clean eggs should be set for incubation because clean eggs hatch better than the soiled eggs. However, dry cleaning of slightly soiled eggs with rough cloth or sand paper may be done before setting but involves considerable risk o explosion in incubator.

7. Transportation of hatching eggs

Eggs which have been shaken or jarred in transit should be allowed to settle for 24 hours or so before setting in incubator.

Factors Affecting Hatchability of Eggs

We have dealt several factors that influence hatching of eggs, such as pre-incubation storage and incubation conditions. In addition, factors, such as egg size, shell quality and age and productivity of breeders have been shown to affect hatchability. A part from these, other factors which influenced hatchability include nutrition of the breeding genetic constitution of the embryo and disease.

a) Nutrition

The egg must contain all the nutrients needed by the embryo, when it is laid by the hen. There is no further contact with the mother once the egg is completed. Therefore, breeder hens must be fed rations that will supply adequate quantities of the nutrients needed for embryo development. Since it is difficult to affect the protein, fat and carbohydrate content of an egg by dietary means, the nutrients most susceptible to diet changes are the vitamins and trace elements.

Nutrient deficiencies can reduce hatchability and often malformed embryos grow as a result of nutrient deficiency. It is difficult to identify the nutrient deficiency responsible for poor hatchability by examination of the embryo. The time of embryo mortality and the deficiency observed often depend on the degree of deficiency of the nutrient involved. Under practical conditions, the nutrients that may reach levels low enough to cause hatchability problems are riboflavin, manganese, pantothenic acid and vitamin B 12 unless some special supplements of these are used.

b) Genetic factors

Genetic factors play a definite role in hatchability of eggs. In breeding has been shown to lower hatchability, whereas it is increased in crossbreds.

c) Diseases

Diseases caused by Salmonella organisms, such as pullorum disease are the major group of bacterial infections that influence hatchability. Salmonella organisms may be passed from infected dams into eggs. The infected eggs as well as non-infected ones do not hatch. Although other disease organisms many not pass into the egg and affect the embryo directly, they may influence the characteristics of the egg and thus indirectly affect its hatchability. Ranikhet disease and infectious bronchitis may affect egg shape and shell porosity. Eggs from hens affected by these diseases frequently do not hatch well because the eggs lose excessive amounts of moisture during incubation. Therefore, hatching eggs from healthy flocks should be selected for incubation.

Hatchability of eggs is of major concern to the hatchery man. There are two independent factors-fertility and hatchability, which affect the production of chicks. Although they are two independent factors, a decrease in either or both of them will reduce the economic returns considerably.

d) Fertility

Some factors are common which affect fertility of both males and females. There are others which affect either of the sexes. For male fertility, the most important consideration is the production of viable spermatozoa capable of fertilising female gametes. There are numerous factors which will influence the semen quality like breed, age of male, nutrition, climatic conditions and method of mating, etc. the female fertility is mainly dependent upon age, method of mating, rate of laying, etc.besides nutritional and climatic factors.

Since optimum fertility is dependent upon both male and female, the important factors involving both of them are the ratio of cock and hens, heredity, system of breeding, etc. If the infertility percentage exceeds 10% some of the above points with respect to fertility should be checked.

e) Male to female ratio

In order to obtain good fertility proper male-female ratio should be maintained. For light breeds 8-10 males for 100 hens and for heavy breeds 12-15 males for 100 hens are adequate.

f) Rate of lay

Rate of egg production influences the frequency of matting and in turn the fertility. Those flocks laying at a high rate usually have a high rate of fertility.

g) Age of males

Breeding males should be at least six or seven months old for resulting in high fertility. Some early sexually maturity strains may fertilise a high percentage of eggs at younger ages, whereas males of slower maturing strains of heavy breeds may not reach to maximum fertility until 8 to 10 months of age.

h) Length of lay

Fertility is higher in first year than the subsequent year. It is also higher in first few months of laying and then declines. It is particularly noticeable in heavy meat type chicken.

i) Weather

Fertility declines considerably during severe hot and cold conditions.

j) Inheritance

Fertility is poorly heritable traits. In addition, fertility is also influenced by nutrition.

Embryonic Development

A study of chick embryology deals with the development of the individual from the origin of the germ cells to the time hatching. Fertilisation of the ovum by the spermatozoa takes place at the upper end of the oviduct probably before albumen is deposited around the yolk. As soon as the male and female cells unite embryonic development beings and continues as long as the incubating temperature is supplied, until the embryo dies or the chick hatches. Thus, the evidence is that embryonic development progresses while the egg is held within the body of the female, and that it continues until the egg is placed in a temperature which holds development in abeyance.

A thorough knowledge of embryonic development of the chick is of great value to those who can apply it in the operation of incubators. It is an aid in securing satisfactory hatches and can be used to check up mistakes in the incubation practice and to rectify them in future changes in chick embryo on day-to-day basis.

First Day : The germinal disc becomes large; part of the yolk around the disc gets darker.

Second Day : Embryo takes definite shape. The tubular heart is formal and its curvature begins. At about 44 hours of incubation, it beats rhythmically. The embryo lies directly across the top of the yolk.

Third Day : Embryo starts to turn over onto left side with top of head towards air cell. Development of the eyes has begun.

Fourth Day : By this time, the body is completely turned onto the left side. Ramifying blood vessels should be clearly evident by this time. Two fetal membranes, namely the amnion and allantois are clearly visible. The allantois serves as temporary lungs.

Fifth Day : The vascular area extends over about two-thirds of the yolk. Limb stocks begin to bend for elbows of wings and the knee of legs. Heart takes on definite shape.

Sixth and Seventh Day : Distinct avian characters are observable, such as the crop, gizzard, caeca, beak and the feather tracts. Obvious movements begin in limbs and amnion (sac in which developing embryo is rocked in the amniotic fluid) .

Eighth, Ninth and Tenth Days : Feather tracts are more distinct and appear along back, neck and thighs. Toes have appeared on the feet and there is a chalky deposit about the mouth, which forms the horny beak.

Eleventh Day : Abdominal walls are definitely established Embryo is nearing completion.

Twelfth and Thirteenth Day : Ossification of the bones well distributed over the body. The cartilaginous skeleton is completed, the nails are visible and the beak is horny but soft. From this time on embryonic development is merely a matter of growth and the complete functioning of all organs.

Fourteenth and Fifteenth Days : The embryo accommodates itself to the long axis of the egg head toward the large end.

Sixteenth Day : The white of the egg is disappearing.

Seventeenth, Eighteenth and Nineteenth Days : The intestine is being drawn into the body cavity. Fluid decreased in the amnion. The neck acquired a double bend so that the head is turned forward, with the beak towards the part of the shell membrane next to the air cell. The chick is now in a hatching position. Yolk sac in beginning to outer the body cavity towards the end of this period.

Twentieth and Twenty First Days : The yolk sac is completely included within the body cavity and practically all of the ammotic fluid has disappeared. The chick now occupies all of the egg outside the air cell and the blood circulation becomes more rapid in the lung tissue. Now the chick raises its head and pierces the shell membrane and slowly breathes the enclosed air. It may then be heard to peep. When the chick pips, the shell, it begins to breathe normally. The function of the allantom is completed; so it rapidly dries up. The chick is now ready to emerge from the shell and complete the hatching process.

Incubation of Chick Embryo by Days

First Day

1. The primitive streak is formed and its axis the primitive groove develops.
2. With the development of the head fold comes the first definite appearance of the head.
3. One or more pairs of somatic make their appearance.
4. The first trace of the amnion appears in front of the head-fold.
5. The vascular area begins to be distinguishable.

Second Day

1. Elevation of the head occurs.
2. The tubular heart and blood vessels form.
3. Eyes appear as hollow birds
4. Auditory pits converted into pockets
5. Head-fold moves backward
6. Curvature of the heart increases
7. Soon after 33 hours, heart begins to twitch at regular intervals, by 44 hours it beats regularly.

Third Day

1. Embryo commences to turn over.
2. Circulation of yolk sac is completed and the curvature of heart is increased.

3. The eye-lens, nerves, etc. are formed.
4. The hind-brain separates into cerebellum and the medulla-oblongata
5. Nasal pits form.
6. The cranial and spinal nerves are established.
7. Formation of fore and hind guts, division of fore-gut into oesophagus, stomach (proventriculus) and gizzard duodenum and later on large intestines.

Fourth Day

1. Great increase in blood circulation in vascular area.
2. Ammonia becomes more conspicuous
3. Tail fold increases
4. Limbs form
5. Olfactory grooves are shaped
6. Absorption of the partition between mouth and throat occurs.
7. The ureter forms
8. Embryo is completely on left side
9. Allantois appears as small pear-shaped vesicle.

Fifth Day

1. Vascular area extends over two-third of the yolk.
2. Allantois is very vascular and serves a chief organ of respiration.
3. Limb stocks begin to bend for elbow and knee; cartridge is formed which proceeds bones in limbs.
4. Heart takes on definite shape.
5. Primitive cartilaginous cranium takes the shape.
6. Parts of the face develop and nasal process close in.
7. Large development of gray matter is noticeable in spinal cord.

Sixth and seventh Days

1. Distinct avian characters are present
2. Crop, caeca and gizzard are visible

3. Nose develops into a beak
4. Obvious movements begin in lambs and amnion. Seventh day amnion pulsates slowly and rhythmically rocking embryo in the amniotic fluid and permits normal development without adhesion.
5. Allantois is much larger
6. Body begins to grow more rapidly in comparison with the head.
7. The egg tooth begins to develop on the sixth day. Its function is for the single critical event breaking of the shell.

Eighth, Ninth and Tenth Days

1. About the 10th day little sacks containing the feathers begin to appear, along back, neck and thighs.
2. Chalky deposit shows about the mouth. It will change into the horny beak.

Eleventh Day

1. Abdominal walls are definitely established. Loops of the intestine which have been hanging in the somatic stock are confined within the cavity of the abdomen.

Twelfth and Thirteenth Days

1. Beak is horny but soft.
2. Nails are visible on 13th day.
3. The cartilaginous skeleton is completed on the 13th day and the various muscles of the body are fairly distinct.
4. Ossification of bones is well distributed over the body

Fourteenth and Fifteenth Days

1. Embryo accommodated itself to the long axis of the eggs, head towards broad end.

Sixteenth to Twenty First Days

1. By the 16th day white of egg has practically disappeared.
2. After 16th day the ureters are abundant in the allantoic fluid.

3. Seventeenth to Nineteenth Days
    a) Fluid decreases in the amnion
    b) The neck acquires a double bend so that the head is turned forward with beak towards the part of the shell membrane next to air cell.
    c) The intestine is retracted completely within the body cavity.
    d) On the 19th day, the yolk sac begins to enter the body cavity.
    e) On the 20th day, the yolk sac is completely included and practically all the amniotic fluid has disappeared.
4. The chick now occupies all the egg outside of the air chamber. The umbilicus is closing over.
5. The blood circulation in the allantois is beginning to contract and more blood is going through the lungs.
6. Now the chick raises its head and pierces the shell membrane and slowly breathes the enclosed air. It may then be heard to peep.
7. Circulation in the allantois is still maintained and it still preserves its respiratory function.

When the chick pips the shell, it begins to breathe normally. The allantois begins to dry up and the circulation in it rapidly ceases. It then becomes separated from the umbilicus and the remainder of the act of hatching is completed.

Functions of fetal membranes

Amnion-Acts as (1) Shock absorber

(2) Protection against desiccation of the embryo

(3) Guard against adhesions

Chorion- Not important in chick development

Allantois- Seroes as embryonic organ of respiration, receiving excretion of the kidneys and absorb the albumen

Yolk sac- Absorbs yolk material

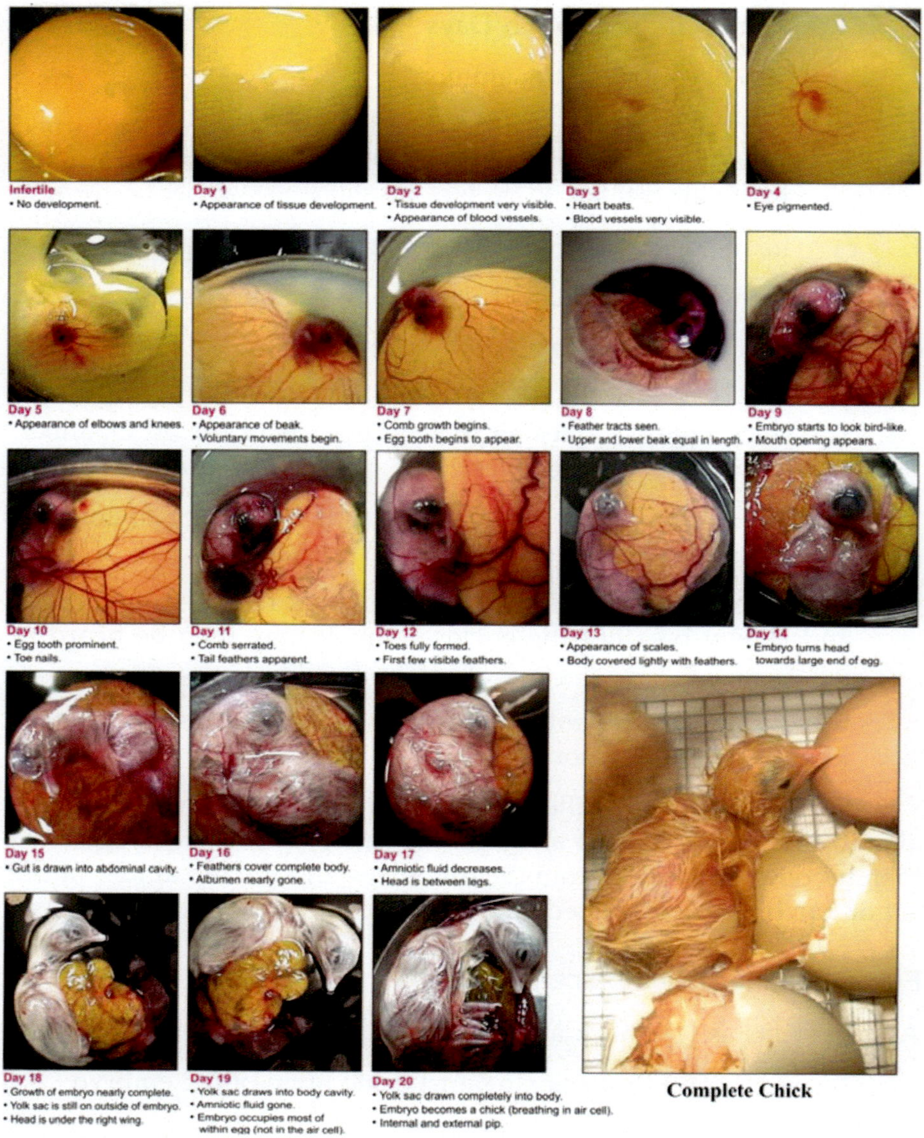

Chick Embryo Development
Source: Desh Biological words, Haryana, India

Malpositions of Embryo

Anyone who makes a careful study and examination of unhatched eggs will readily mote that there are a number of abnormalities, which are so severe as to result in the failure of many embryos to hatch.

Normally, a chick ready to hatch lies with its head in the large end of the egg, its legs towards the small end, the head turned to the right and lying under the right wing, with the beak directed towards the air cell.

The fundamental causes of the defective condition in an embryo, whether they be from the effects of inbreeding, of faulty nutrition, or of careless incubation methods will interfere with the normal sequence of body shiftings and as a consequence will leave the embryo in a retarded or strained position, when death occurs. The following are the different malpositions in an egg:

Table 3: Different malpositions in an egg

Position No.	Description
i)	Head between thighs
ii)	Head in small end
iii)	Head to left instead of under right wing
iv)	Head normal, but rotated away from air cell
v)	Feet over head
vi)	Beak over right wing or over and under wing

It has been shown that the frequency of Position IV is reduced, when the eggs are incubated with the large end up. Unfortunately, however, the large-end-up position causes an increase in the number of malpositions I and II. Position III is markedly more frequent in the larger eggs.

Sexing of chicks

There are two methods of chick sexing as:

1. Vent method : It is very popular and originally developed in Japan. It depends upon the observation of rudimentary sex organ. In case of males, there are three bean-shaped bumps, whereas in females centre prolurberance is missing. Chick sexing machine is also available which is a tube like structure having magnifying lens and eye lens to see through. It enlarges the view of sex organs by 3-5 times. However, the disadvantage with this machine is that the sexing process is slower than the one with naked eye.
2. In-auto-sexing : Plumage colour linked with sex chromosome is taken into account to determine the sex. When a Rhode Island

Red male is mated to Barred Plymouth rock female, all the female progeny will be black and male progeny barred.

Grading day old chicks

The chicks below the minimum standards should not be allowed to go to the customers. Some standards for chick quality are:

a) No. of chick deformities

b) No. of chick navels

c) Above a minimum weight

d) Not dehydrated

e) Down colour representative of the breed

f) Stand up well

Diagnosis of hatch failure : Eggs failed to hatch can be judged and examining them for certain diagnostic signs based on the appearance and comparative development of the egg and embryo. Break the egg into a flat container and evaluate the contents according to the following criteria:

Clears : Absence of a blood ring or embryo developed indicates that either the embryo died early in incubation or the eggs were infertile.

Blood rings : Clear eggs with a blood-ring or small embryo indicate that death occurred in the first three days of incubation possibly because of incubators malfunction.

Early-dead or mid-term embryo : Possible causes include excessively high or low incubator temperatures, improper turning, low viability of the egg caused by parental nutrition or inheritance, improper ventilation and suffocation, disease, poor egg shell quality and contamination.

Fully formed and not piped : The usual causes include low average incubation temperature, weak viability of setting eggs, improper humidity, genetic defects, contamination or temperature malfunction.

Malformed chicks : Genetic deformities may occur. High temperature during certain formation times may lead to deformities. Rough handling of incubating eggs may contribute to malformation.

Trouble shooting hatch failures : Eggs do not hatch for reasons which may or may not be the fault of the person caring for the eggs.

Below are few common reasons for incubation failures

Infertile eggs: Procure the fertile hatching eggs from farms having at least one male with every ten females.

Parent stock : Weak and unhealthy or nutritionally deficient diet fed parent stock. The care for breeder flock should be taken following sound poultry management practices.

Eggs are too old or improperly cared for before incubation

The following hatching eggs should not be stored for longer than 7-10 days before incubation.

Shell contamination

Incubate only clean or slightly dirty eggs cleaned with sandpaper. Do not wash dirty hatching eggs or allow eggs to sweat before placing them in the incubator.

Temperature too high, too low or too variable

Check incubator temperature with an accurate thermometer and adjust the thermostat accordingly.

Too little or too much humidity in the incubator

Obtain a hygrometer and measure the humidity before making further adjustments.

Eggs not turned often enough

Turn eggs at least two or three times daily. Commercial hatcheries turn eggs every two hours.

Improper ventilation resulting in low oxygen

Forced-air incubators should start with vent opening half opened. Increase ventilation after ten days until openings are fully opened at hatching time.

Rough handling of eggs

Excessive handling and jarring of eggs while turning especially during the first week may be harmful.

Breakout Analysis

A breakout analysis of hatching eggs must be done to evaluate the breeder flocks progress with respect to fertility and hatchability. It is an absolutely essential diagnostic tool for identifying the cause(c) of problems in hatchability. These are of three types: (1) Breakout of fresh, non-incubated eggs; (2) breakout of incubated (5 to 12d) eggs and (3) Breakout of eggs that did not hatch (hatch residue).

For breakout analysis eggs should be removed from the setter/hatcher tray, placed on egg flats and identified as per the flock, location, etc. The exterior of the egg is examined first for eggs traits, piping and location of the air cell. The shell is cracked at the large end, over the air cell and a hole opened in the hell and membranes to observe the interior of the egg. If the egg appears to be infertile or contains a very early dead embryo, the germinal disc must be located to make a definite identification of fertility. If the embryo is relatively small, the egg can be broken into a dish for further examination. Eggs with late-stage embryos should be observed for pipping into the air cell, and then opened with scissors from large end to small end without disturbing the position of embryo. The embryos position, the embryos age, malformations, contamination and other factors should be observed and recorded. Comparisons will live embryos of various ages can be done to train those developing experience in the breakout technique.

Breakout of fresh eggs is used to provide an immediate evaluation of flock fertility. The breakout following candling will include eggs determined to the infertile, eggs containing early dead and cracked eggs. The hatch residue breakout includes all eggs that did not hatch. Candle breakout and residue breakout should be done weekly or at least every 3 weeks. Regular, consistent analysis of these breakouts will result in flock histories that can be used to diagnose hatchability problems, minimize losses, and compare strains, flocks, farms, hatcheries and many other variables.

Table 4: A diagnosis chart to assist in solving incubation failures

Symptoms	Probable Cause	Corrective Measures
Clear eggs with no embryonic development (Infertile eggs)	Eggs damaged by environment Eggs stored too long or incorrectly	Gather eggs frequently (at least once daily) Store eggs at 50-60^{0}F and 60% relative humidity. Incubate eggs within 7 days of lay.
Blood rings	Improper storage Improper incubation temperature Improper fumigation	Follow recommend egg storage and collection recommendations. Check thermometer accuracy and incubation functions. Follow fumigation recommendation.
Many dead embryos at early stages	Improper incubation temperatures (Usually too high) Improper egg turning Improper ventilation	Follow recommend incubation temperatures. Turn at least 3 times daily Increase ventilation rate in incubator and/or room, but avoid drafts.
Early hatching (may have haemorrhagic navels)	Pullorum disease High incubation temperatures	Use eggs from disease-free sources. Have blood-test of the breeder flock. Follow recommended incubation temperatures. Check equipment for proper function. Guard against electrical surges or high incubator room temperatures.
Late hatching or not hatching uniformly	Improper storage Low incubation temperatures Warm and cool spots in incubator due to faulty design Old or improperly stored eggs	Store eggs at 50-60^{0}F and 60% RH. Turn at least 3 times daily. Follow recommend incubation temperatures contact incubator company or obtain a different incubator design. Gather eggs frequently, cool immediately and store eggs properly. Do not store longer than 7 days.
Sticky embryos (Embryos may be smeared with egg contents)	High average incubation humidity Inadequate ventilation	Follow recommend incubation humidity heck size of air cell as an indicator for adjusting humidity condition.

		Increase ventilation rate in incubator and or room, but avoid drafts.
Embryos sticking or adhering to shell	Improper incubation temperature (usually too high Low incubation humidity Improper egg setting positions or turning during incubation. Slick hatching trays	Follow recommend incubation temperatures. Increase incubation humidity by increasing water evaporation. Set eggs with small end down. Turn eggs at least 3 times daily. Do not turn eggs within 3 days of hatching. Use trays with wire floors or place crinoline on hatching surface.
Large, soft-bodied mushy chicks dead on trays; bad odour	Low average incubation temperature Poor ventilation Naval infection (omphatitis)	Follow recommended incubation temperatures Increase ventilation rate in incubator and/or room, but avoid drafts. Clean and disinfect incubators and hatching units between settings of eggs. Maintain dry hatching trays. Properly store and fumigate eggs.
Rough or unhealed navels	Improper incubation temperatures High hatching humidity Naval infection (omphatitits)	Follow recommend incubation temperatures Maintain proper humidity. Clean and disinfect incubator and hatching ubits between settings of eggs. Maintain dry hatching trays. Properly store and fumigate eggs.

Hatchery Hygiene and Fumigation

The hatchery must always be regarded as the greatest potential source from where diseases can spread. There are two classes of diseases which originate from hatchery. The first includes those diseases which are definitely egg transmittable. The second includes diseases that are transmitted by contact with disease producing micro-organism introduced from sources other than eggs after the chiks are hatched. Examples of first group are Pullorum disease and Salmonellosis and the examples of second group are: Omphatitis, Ranikhet disease and the respiratory diseases.

Table 5: Diseases affecting hatchability and chick quality

Pullorum Disease	Infectious Bronchitis
Arizona Disease	New castle Disease
Fowl Typhoid	Avian Encephalonylitis
Paralyphoid	Mycoplasma gallisepticin
Aspergillosis	Mycoplasma
Omphatitis	Mycoplasma synoviae
Eschercia Coli	Laryngotrachitis

Prevention of egg borne diseases is best effected by using eggs from disease free flocks. Prevention of the second group depends largely on the standard of sanitation maintained especially in the hatchery.

Fumigation

It has been reported that organisms causing Pullorum, paralyphoid, infectious Coryza and Omphalitis and the viruses of infectious Laryngotracheitis. Infectious Bronchitis, Fowl Pox and Ranikhet Disease (ND) can be effectively destroyed by fumigation.

When to fumigate

A desirable practice is to fumigate the incubator between hatches. In case of separate hatchers, fumigation can be done after each hatch but in case of combined incubation and hatching compartments, fumigation should be taken up at the designing of incubation of incubation and also in between hatches. Fumigation during the incubation period should not ordinarily be practical, which may lower hatchability.

Method of fumigation

Fumigation is accomplished by the use of formaldehyde gas, which may either be liberated from a chemical reaction or simply released from an aqueous suspension. Accordingly, there are two methjods of fumigation :

a) Potassium permanganate method

b) Cheese cloth method

Before fumigation, it is necessary to know the cubic space inside the incubator, which is obtained by multiplying the height, width and depth of the incubator, with a view to determine the optimum quantity of chemical required. The incubator is then operated in the normal way, maintaining the usual temperature nbut slightly higher humidity as during hatching. Fumigation is carried out only after the required temperature and humidity has been attained.

a) Potassium permanganate method : Crystals of potassium permanganate are taken in a shallow-pan and placed near the fan in the incubator, then commercial formalin is added to it and door closed for 3 hours while the incubator is running. The quantity of potassium permanganate required is 15 grams and formalin 30 ml. for every 100 cubic feet of incubator space. The chemical reaction between the two results in the liberation of formaldehyde gas which accomplishes fumigation. In some cases much stronger fumigation, such as double strength or triple strength fumigation is used by increasing the quantity of chemicals by two or three-fold.

Table 6: Concentration and duration of formaldehyde fumigation required

Period	Concentration	Time (Min)
Hatching eggs, soon after lay	3x	20
Eggs in Incubator (First day)	2x	20
Chicks in hatcher	1x	3
Incubator room	1x, 2x	30
Hatcher, between hatches	3x	30
Hatcher room chick room between hatches	3x	30
Chick boxes, pads, poultry equipments	3x	30
Trucks	5x	20

b) Cheese cloth method: In this method, cheese cloth or muslin cloth of about one square yard size is taken and immersed in sufficient quantity of commercial formalin to supply 20 ml. for every 100 ft. of incubator space. The formalin soaked cloth is then hug in the incubator close to the fan. The incubator door is closed and fumigation done for 3 hours while the incubator keeps operating.

❑❑❑

Chapter 5

Systems of Poultry Farming

Poultry farming is practiced under a wide range of conditions, which can be classified into one of the following broad farming systems:

i) Extensive system (Free-range extensive and Backyard extensive systems)

ii) Semi-intensive system, and

iii) Intensive system.

In earlier days, poultry were primarily reared as backyard unit. They used to be scavenging in the morning hours and by the evening they return home to be kept under a night shelter with some water and left-over food or grains. These birds are hardly and no expense is involved in the rearing of such birds. However, they produce less number of eggs and meat. Under emergency, they can be easily sold. The system of rearing birds under these conditions is broadly called as extensive poultry farming system. But as the scientists improved the efficiency of the birds to produce more eggs and meat, the needs of the birds also increased. As the ability of the birds improved, their requirements also increased in terms of housing, feeding, breeding, healthcare and overall management. The systems of rearing birds under these improved conditions are broadly called as semi-intensive or intensive poultry farming system. The system of housing being practiced by the poultry farmers is the broad basis for the classification of extensive/semi-extensive or semi-intensive/intensive poultry farming.

Extensive System

Under free-range extensive system, the birds are not confined and can scavenge for food over a wide area. Rudimentary shelters may or may not be provided to the birds, and these may or may not be used. The birds may roost outside, usually in trees, and nest in the bushes. The flock may comprise birds of different species and varying ages.

They are usually fed a handful of grain in the morning and evening to supplement scavenging.

Many local *(Desi)* birds are being reared in our country in this way. Most of these birds are reared for hobby and whatever is obtained from them is taken as bonus. In each unit, the number of birds reared will be limited to a maximum of 10 to 15.

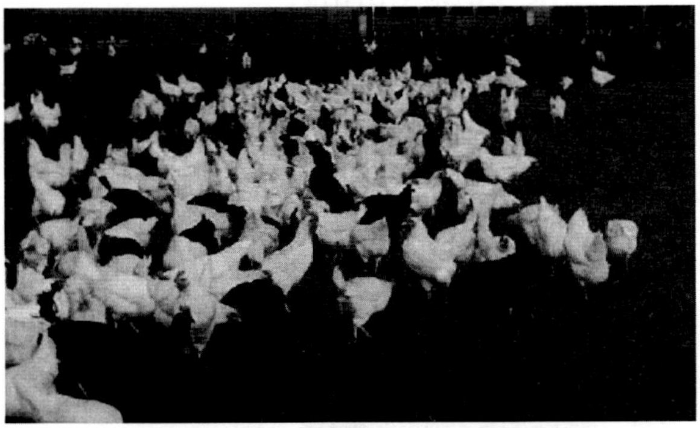

Extensive system of rearing poultry

i) Advantages

- No need of a separate house for the birds.
- No need of a balanced feeding because they graze and eat outside.
- Cost on feeding is virtually negligible since only left-over feed or grains will be given to the birds.
- As the birds are exposed to sunshine, they can produce their own Vitamin D.

ii) Disadvantages

- Birds are likely to be eaten away by predators like dogs, eagles, etc.
- There can be losses due to theft.
- They are exposed to all diseases; some of them can spread to humans also. More likely to have parasites both inside (endo-parasite) and on the body (ecto-parasite).
- They may not get proper food.
- Due to above factors, they produce very few eggs; say about 50 to 60 in a year.

- They weigh very less; about 1.0 to 1.2 kg, when they are sold after 18 months of age.

Semi-intensive System

It is also called semi-extensive system. This system consists of a separate shelter for the birds during the night in which water and some feed is provided. Litter material is spread on the floor. This shelter will be fenced all round giving sufficient area for the birds to graze during the day. Obviously, area available for grazing depends on the land covered by the fence. However, this system is popular for rearing turkeys and ducks than chicken. In case of ducks, a pond for them to swim may also be provided.

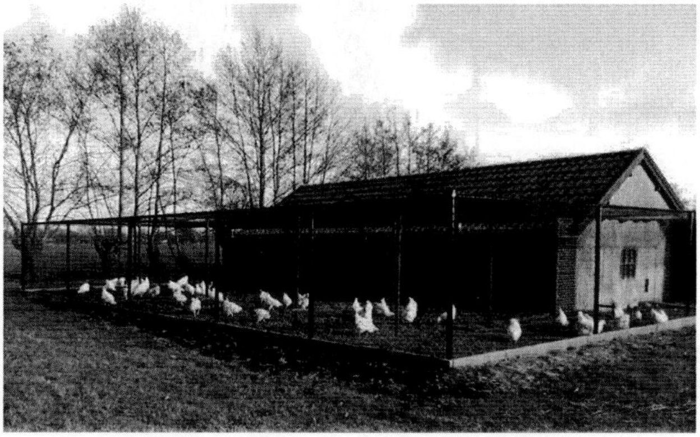

Semi-intensive system of housing poultry

i) Advantages

- Birds need some care at least during the night.
- Even during the day, due to fencing, chances of theft are also minimized.
- Fencing also limits predator attacks and diseases.
- As the birds are exposed to sunshine, they can produce their own Vitamin D.

ii) Disadvantages

- Requires more land.
- Predator attacks are not totally restricted.
- Losses due to theft also are not eliminated due to fencing alone.

- Unless specific vaccination program is followed, the birds are also exposed to diseases. They are also more likely to have parasites both inside and on the body.
- They may not get proper food, because only during night, some feed is given, which need not be a standard one.
- They also produce very few eggs; say about 50 to 60 in a year with less weight.

Intensive system

Due to improvements in the ability of birds to grow and produce, extensive and semi- intensive systems are not commercially practiced in our country. The word "Intensive" means more concentrated or more numbers per unit area or more intensity. Therefore, in all the systems under this category, more birds can be reared in a given area than in semi-intensive or extensive systems. They are restricted into a house where they are provided food, water and all other requirements. Therefore, intensive system can also be called 'in-house system' or water.

In the intensive system of rearing poultry, the following are practiced:

- Deep litter system
- Cage system
- Slat system
- Alternate system

In India, deep litter and cage systems are more popular and mostly practiced.

Deep Litter System

In this system, birds are left free on the floor. To avoid cleaning of the floor everyday, a soft bedding material is spread on the floor which can absorb moisture on the floor. This material is called as "Litter material". It forms very good manure. Since the litter becomes deeper day-by-day, the system is referred to as "Deep litter system". Birds do scratch and peck in the litter and even get certain vitamins and unknown growth factors while doing so! Most of the broilers in India are being reared under this system.

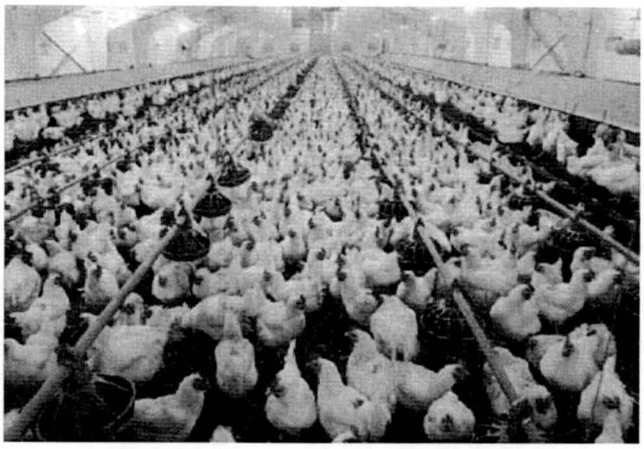

Deep litter system of rearing poultry

Characteristics of Good Litter Material : A good litter material should:

- Be light in weight
- Be fairly coarse to prevent caking
- Be highly absorbent
- Dry rapidly by releasing absorbed moisture into the incoming air
- Be soft and compressible
- Be cheap
- Form part of the manure
- Be easily available during all times of the year

Commonly Used Litter Materials

Paddy straw, ground nut shells, wood shavings, maize cobs, maize straw, etc. can be used as litter materials and paddy straw is by far the most commonly employed one.

Advantages

- Deep-litter keeps cool during summer and warm during winter. Hence, the birds will be comfortable during all seasons.
- They can move freely, also adds to their comfort.
- Birds derive certain un-identified growth factors.
- There will be no incidence of swellings or damaged breast region in case of broilers.

- Usually, there will be no problem of ammonia accumulation and house-flies in a well-managed deep-litter flock.
- Incidence of broken eggs is very minimal.
- There will be no problem of caged layer fatigue.
- There will be uniform distribution of light in the layer house.
- Initial investment is less, when the land cost is low.

Disadvantages

- Less number of birds can be housed in the same space than in cage system.
- Building dimension will be higher than cage system. Therefore, cost of construction of building increases.
- There will be more feed wastage due to spilling from feeding trough.
- Birds consume more feed since they move about more freely wasting some energy.
- Litter-borne diseases especially coccidiosis can occur,.
- Diseases spread faster due to free movement.
- Cannibalism (pecking and eating), if starts, will be severe, when compared to cage system.
- More number of unclean or dirty eggs are produced.
- Birds consume more feed per dozen eggs.
- Broodiness (sitting on eggs to hatch) can be a problem.
- Nests have to be provided and the eggs have to be collected regularly.
- There is a chance of egg-eating vice, especially when the eggs are left in nest boxes or on floor for a long time.
- Fighting among birds is possible.
- Requires more labour than cage system.

Cage System

Increase in cost of land and availability and wages of labour has made litter system costly. Therefore, alternate systems in which birds are totally restricted to meshwork compartments (cages) were introduced. This saves the cost of litter material, reduces labour requirement and building cost. Most of the layers are grown in cages all over the world.

Cages suitable for all age and types of chicken are available. But, in our country, cages are popularly used for layers, whereas others are generally reared on deep litter. Even in cages for layers, 3- bird cages are more popular than 1, 2, 4, 15 or 30-bird cages. Cages housing 15 or 30 hens are popularly called "Community or Colony cages".

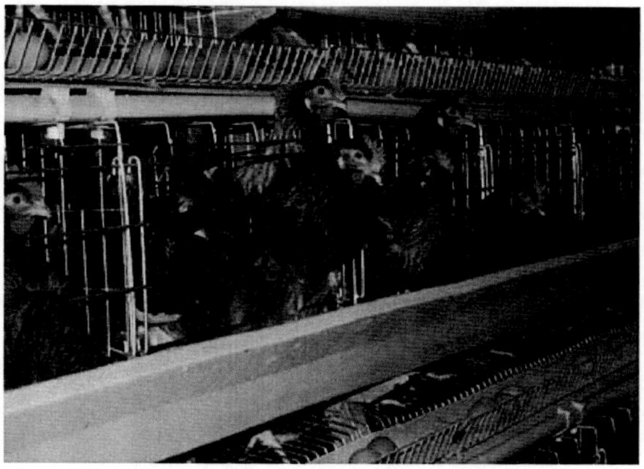

Cage system of housing

a) Advantages

- This system can accommodate more number of birds in a given space than any other system.
- Movement of birds is restricted and hence, they consume less feed when compared to other systems.
- There will be less wastage of feed because movement is restricted.
- No problem of litter-borne diseases, especially coccidiosis.
- Spread of disease is slower than other systems.
- Incidence of cannibalism is minimum.
- Birds lay more and heavier eggs.
- Consume less feed per dozen eggs produced.
- Eggs will be cleaner than in other systems.
- Broodiness is avoided.
- Labour requirement is minimum.

b) Disadvantages

- Birds are uncomfortable because they are not able to move freely.
- Birds suffer from boredom. It is common to fix a coloured plastic wheel in all cages so that the birds can peck at them and play; but it cannot substitute for free movement and association between birds.
- During summer, birds are most uncomfortable due to high temperature. If humidity also is high as is expected in coastal places, so the birds feel very uncomfortable.

Different Species Involved Under Poultry Farming

1. Chicken Farming

Under chicken farming, a farmer may opt for starting either:

- Broiler farming for meat
- Layer farming - for eggs (table and hatching eggs), production of replacement pullets and chick production.

Besides the nutritive value, eggs have many industrial uses in preparation of adhesives, printer inks, shampoos, soap, varnishes, vaccines, etc. The egg shells are used as mineral-feed for animals and birds. The feathers are used for making various goods, such as cushions, mattresses, pillows, etc.

Farmers can rear the birds under free range (extensive), semi-intensive, and intensive (deep litter/cage) systems.

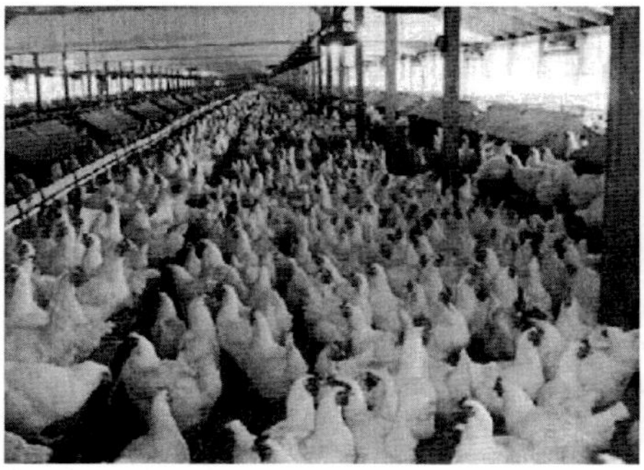
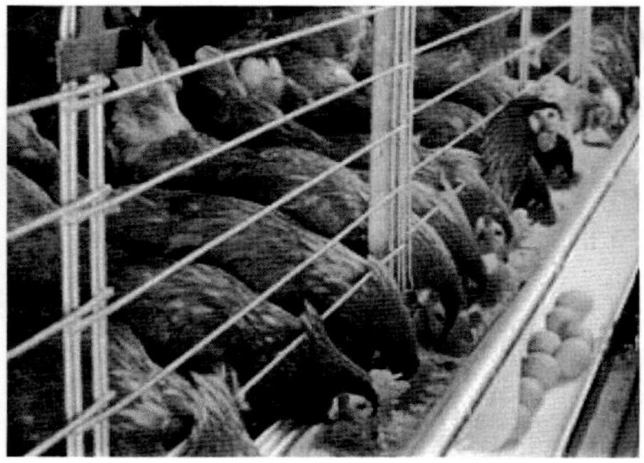

Chicken farming in deep litter and cage systems

Classification of chicken

a) **Based on the place of origin**

- **Asiatic :** Brahma, Langshan, Cochin
- **American :** Plymouth Rock, Rhode Island Red, Wyandotte
- **Mediterranean :** Leghorn, Minorca, Ancona
- **English :** Orpington , Sussex, Cornish

b) **Based on utility, economics or commercial value**

- **Egg-type** *:* e.g. Leghorn
- **Meat-type** *:* e.g. Cornish, Plymouth Rock
- **Dual purpose** *:* e.g. Rhode Island Red, New Hampshire
- **Game type** *:* e.g. Aseel.

General characteristics of various classes of chicken

American Class

- Body size - Medium to heavy
- Egg shell colour -Brown
- Shanks- Clean and yellow, Skin - yellow (except Jersey Black giant, where the shanks are black) Earlobes-Red
- Comb Shape- Rose or Single
- Eg. Plymouth rock, Wyandotte, Rhode Island Red, Jersey Black giant, New Hampshire

Asiatic Class

- Body size -Heavy
- Egg shell colour-Brown,
- Broody with motherly instinct
- Earlobes -Red, mostly
- Shank - feathered and yellow
- Skin - Yellow (except Langshan)
- e.g: Brahma, Cochin, Langshan

English Class

- Body size - Medium to large
- Egg shell colour - Brown
- Earlobes - Red
- Shank - Clean and White
- Skin -White
- Comb shape -Single (except Cornish with pea comb)
- e.g: Australorp, Cornish, Dorking, Orpington and Sussex

Mediterranean Class

- Body size -Small
- Egg-type, non-broody
- Egg shell colour - White
- Ear lobes -White
- Shanks - Clean and Yellow/slate coloured
- Skin -Yellow or White
- e.g: Leghorn, Minorca, Ancona, Andalusian

Table 1: Indigenous chicken of india

Bred (Origin/ Breeding tract)	Varieties
Aseel (Andhra Pradesh, Uttar Pradesh, Rajasthan)	Nhurie (white), Peela (golden yellow), Khagar (black), Yakuth (black and red), Chitta (black and white), Subja (white and golden), Reza (light red).
Kadaknath (Madhya Pradesh)	
Bursa (Gujarat, Maharashtra)	
Chittagong/Malay (Chittagong hills)	
Naked neck (Maharashtra)	
Ankleshwar (Gujarat)	
Kashmir Favorella (Kashmir)	
Denki (Odisha)	

Hybrids of chicken

- These are incrossbreds of poultry, produced by 2-way, 3-way or 4-way crossing of inbred pure lines.
- They are the actual commercial-type of poultry used for egg or meat production; since they are high laying/fast growing. However, they will not breed-true and are unfit for further breeding.
- These birds possess high degree of heterosis and hybrid vigour.

1. Common egg-type hybrid chicken

- BV-300, ISA, Babcock, Bovans, Euribrid, Hyline, HH-260, Dekalb, Keystone, Lohmann and H & N Nick chick.

2. Common Meat-type hybrid chicken

- Cobb, Ross, Steggles, Arbor acres, Hub chicks, Hybro, Hubbard, Lohmann, Pilch, Starbro, Tegel, Anak-2000, Marshall, Peterson, Samrat-2000 and Avian-34.

2. Duck Farming

The ducks occupy second place to chicken in population in the country. They are reared mainly for egg and meat purposes. Duck production is mostly concentrated in the eastern and southern states like Assam, Manipur, Tripura and West Bengal followed by Andhra Pradesh, Bihar, Jammu and Kashmir, Karnataka, Kerala, Odisha, Tamil Nadu, and Uttar Pradesh.

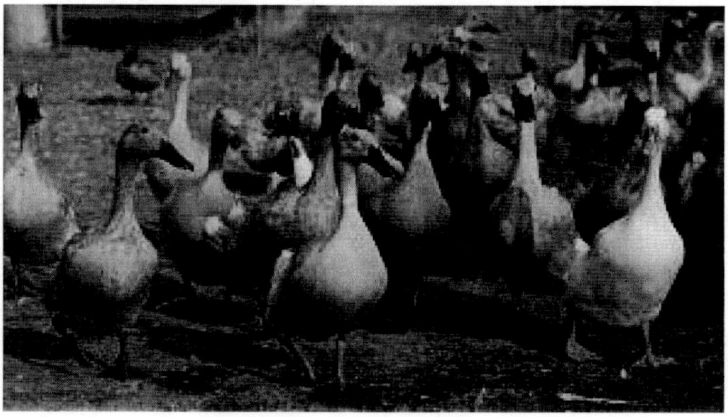

Duck farming

The duck rearing is more popular due to the following advantages:

- Availability of ponds and waterways as Chickens do not flourish in marshy wetland area, which are ideal for duck rearing.
- These watershed areas in addition to lakes and ponds provide algae, earthworms, fungi, insects, small fishes, snails, water weeds, etc., as natural food for the ducks and thus reduce the feed cost.
- Ducks lay about 160-180 eggs in a year.
- Ducks also enrich the soil by their droppings while foraging.
- Duck eggs are heavier by 15-20 grams than chicken eggs.
- Requires less care and attention in management.
- Comparatively, ducks are more resistant to diseases than chicken.
- Majority of ducks lays eggs before 9.00 A.M. which helps in easy egg collection as well as saves labour cost.
- Acts as biological vector and control many diseases by destroying snails.
- Suitable for mixed farming system, such as duck-cum-fish farming.

The domesticated breeds of ducks can be classified as follows:

- Egg type breeds
- Meat type breeds
- Ornamental type breeds and
- Indigenous breeds

A) Egg type breeds

Campbell

- Campbell ducks - developed by Mrs. Campbell during the beginning of the 19th century by crossing Rouen (male line) with Indian Runner (female line)
- Khaki Campbell is a variety resulted from colour selection of the Campbell breed

Indian Runner - derives its name from its place of introduction- East India.

- The body shape and carriage (posture) resemble the penguins
- Three standard varieties - Fawn, White and White penciled
- They are excellent layers and thus, formed the female line in developing the Campbell ducks

Nageswari

- It is an indigenous egg type breed of duck commonly seen in North-eastern part of the country.
- These birds are highly resistant to disease and capable of laying 180-200 eggs even under the range system of rearing.
- The females weigh around 1.5 kg and males weighing 1.7 kg.

B) Meat type breeds

Pekin - These ducks originated in China

- White Pekin is the most popular duck.The plumage is creamy white, the flesh is yellow and the bill and legs are deep orange
- The adult body weight of drake and duck will be 4 kg and 3 kg
- Early maturity, fleshing and good laying capacity are the special features of this breed
- **Aylesbury -**Native of England
- The plumage colour is spotless white in both the sexes. The legs and feet are orange. It is larger than pekin and the adult drake and duck weigh around 4.5 kg and 4 kg, respectively
- **Rouen ducks -** Originated in France. This formed the basis (male line) for developing Campbell ducks
- **Muscovy** - Originated in South America. The males have no characteristic drake feathers. However, have a knob on the head like a crest. If Muscovy is crossed with other ducks, the progeny will be "sterile" called Mule ducks having high growth rate and lean meat. The incubation period is 35 days.

The plumage colour is spotless white in both the sexes. The legs and feet are orange. It is larger than pekin and the adult drake and duck weigh around 4.5 kg and 4 kg, respectively.

C) Ornamental type

- Buff Orpington, Mandarin, Crested white, etc.

Indigenous duck breeds

- Sythetmet, Nageswari ducks of North-Eastern states
- Kuttanad ducks of Kerala (Variety-Chara and Chemballi)
- Arani ducks of Tamil Nadu

In India, 90-95 per cent of ducks are indigenous or non-descript types, which are hardy, with mediocre egg production and highly suitable for extensive system of rearing.

Hybrid Ducks

- Cherry valley (Both Meat and Egg type)
- Hytop (Mule duck)
- Legarth (Meat-type)

3. Geese Farming

Male geese are known as gander and the females are called geese. In India, the Brown-backed and White geese are found. Some of the specific advantages of geese farming are as follows:

- Hardy and can easily adapt to different feeding and management conditions.
- Have the ability to digest 40-50 % crude fibre; as such, the feed cost can be reduced by incorporating large quantities of high-fibre containing forages in the feed.
- Geese meat has high caloric value.
- Goosling (young geese) can attain a weight of 5 kg at 8 weeks of age with the feed conversion efficiency of about 3.0 kg.

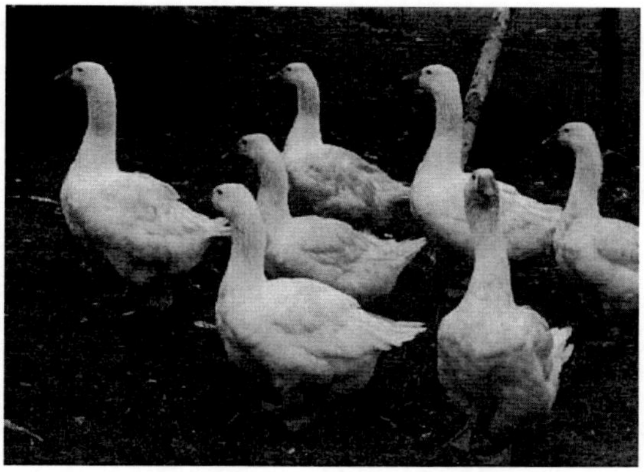

Geese farming

Breeds

Toulouse

- Originated in France. Some strains are non-broody and the goose is a fair layer among the heavy breeds
- Goslings tend to grow slowly and have to be kept to an older age before being ready for market
- The progeny of a Toulouse goose crossed with an Emden gander grows rapidly and has good fleshing qualities Gander-14 kg; Goose-9 kg

Emden

- Originated from Hanover in Germany
- It is a heavy breed, a prolific breeder with a quiet disposition and currently the most popular in New South Wales
- Gooslings can be sexed at day old with a reasonable degree of accuracy as female chicks have a darker down than male chicks
- Bill, legs and feet are bright orange and the hard tight plumage is pure glossy white
- Other goose breeds are African, Chinese, Egyptian, Canada, etc. **Indigenous breed:** Kashmir Anz.

4. Guinea Fowl Farming

India has a large population of guinea fowl and ranks third after chicken and duck. It is well-adapted to diverse agro-climatic conditions prevailing in arid and semi-arid regions and also well accepted by the marginal farmers as well as other vulnerable groups, such as small-scale poultry enterprises raised under free-range in the states of Madhya Pradesh, Punjab, Uttar Pradesh and some parts of India. Lavender, Pearl and White are the three commonly known varieties of guinea fowl in India. The advantages of guinea fowl farming are:

- They are hardy, disease resistant, need low input and has unique ability to survive and thrive under sub-optimal management and feeding conditions because of its foraging habit.
- Meat is tender but pinkish red or dark in colour and having flavour of game bird.
- They are Seasonal breeder and lay eggs between March and September.
- The production starts by 30 weeks of age and lays 130-170 eggs in the first years. The average egg weight is 43-48 g.
- They are highly resistant to viral diseases and therefore, they are generally raised without any vaccination.

Varieties : Pearl, White and Lavender.

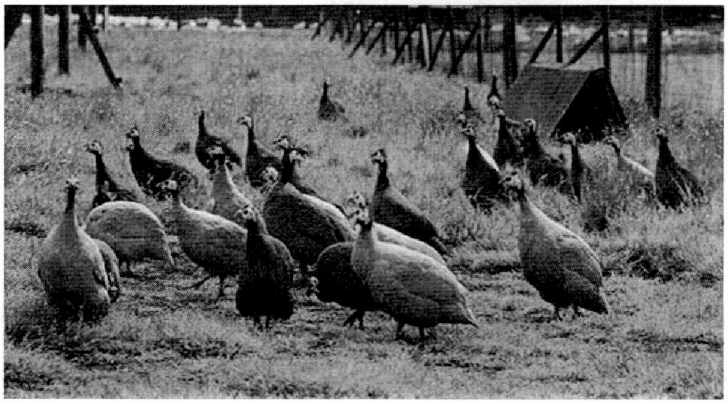

Guinea fowl farming

5. Quail Farming

Japanese quail is mostly reared in India for meat and eggs. The reasons for popularity of quail farming are as follows:

- They are Hardy and it can adapt to various environments.
- They do not require specially designed house.
- They are Fast growing birds, mature in about six weeks and are usually in full production by about seven weeks of age. The live

weight of mature bird is 120-150 g for male and 150-180 g for female.

- They are Prolific layers produce three to four generations per year and lay 260 eggs in their first year of laying.
- The adult quail consumes 20 to 25 g of feed per day and egg weight is 10 to 12 g
- They need less floor, feeder and water space in comparison to chicken and ducks.
- They are more resistant to diseases than chickens.
- They require less capital investment.

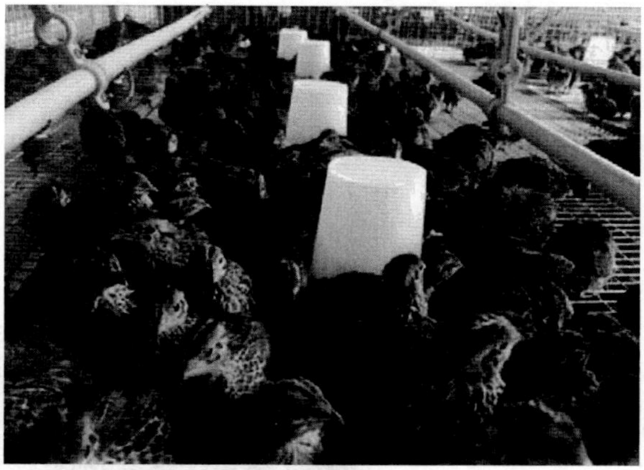

Quail farming

Breeds : Manchurian Golden, British Range, English White and Tuxedo.

6. Turkey Farming

Turkey farming is mostly reared for meat purpose. In India, turkey production is still in its initial stage. Since the turkey hens are bigger in size, their cut-ups can be marketed in various attractive packaging suited to the individual consumer. They are more resistant to disease than chicken and therefore, rarely suffer from diseases. The turkey farming has the following benefits:

- Grows very fast.
- Can be reared under semi-intensive system in the backyards.
- Turkey egg weighs 1.3 times more than the chicken egg.

- More resistant to diseases than the chickens.
- Better forager than chickens.
- Turkey meat contains very less fat when compared to meat of other avian species.

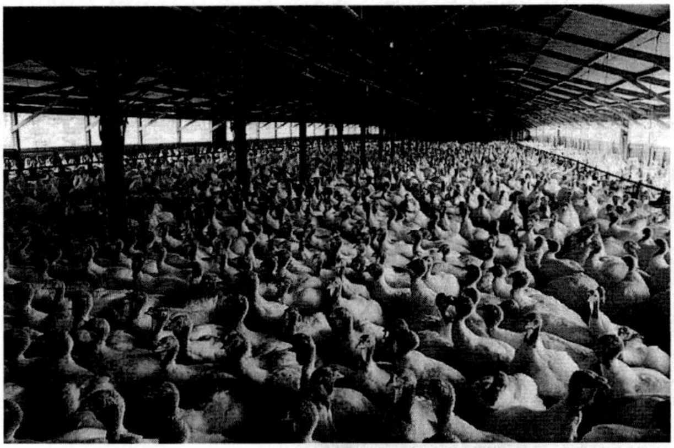

Turkey farming

Common varieties of turkeys

- Broad Breasted Bronze
- Broad Breasted White
- BeltsVille White
- White Holland
- Narragansett

7. Emu Farming

The emu is another latest addition to poultry species for commercial use. The body weight of an adult emu is about 50-60 kg and their height is around 1.70-1.95 meters and out of which least 35 kg of fresh meat can be extracted. Emu meat costs around Rs. 550-600 a kilo. Emu chicks cost more than Rs. 1,500 and bigger birds cost Rs.7,000 to 9,000 depending upon their weight. The birds lay eggs every three days in winter. Its egg weight is 0.7 to 1 kg. Areas, where water is available in abundance, are the best places for emu farming, which is not labour-intensive. The following are the advantages of Emu farming:

- Emu meat contains low amount of fat and cholesterol.
- Emu oil is also estimated to be highly medicinal value and is gaining its popularity in the pharmaceutical industry.
- Colourful Emu eggs are used for ornamental purposes.
- Emu birds are practically immune to several diseases.

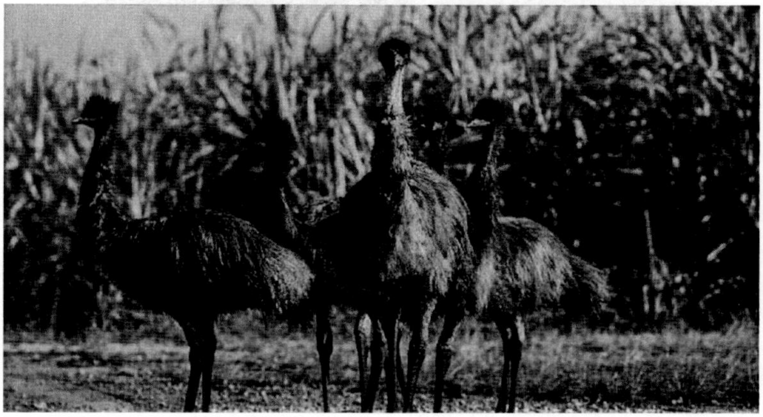

Emu farming

8. Ostrich Farming

Ostrich farming is comparatively a new agribusiness idea compared to other poultry birds. Now-a-days, many countries around the world have started ostrich farming as a new business venture. The Scientific name of ostrich is *'Struthio Camelis'*.

- The feather of ostrich is extremely valuable, which is mainly used for home decoration purposes.
- Their skin is also very valuable, and their meat is considered as very delicious food and has high demand in the international market.
- Ostrich is the biggest bird among all the bird species.
- They also produce the largest eggs.
- An adult male ostrich weights between 63 to 130 kg (140-290 lbs) and an adult female ostrich weights about 155 kg (340 lbs).
- Adult male ostrich feathers are black coloured, primary and caudal feathers are white coloured.

- Female and baby ostrich feather can be of grey or white coloured.
- The neck of the both male and female ostrich is almost featherless.

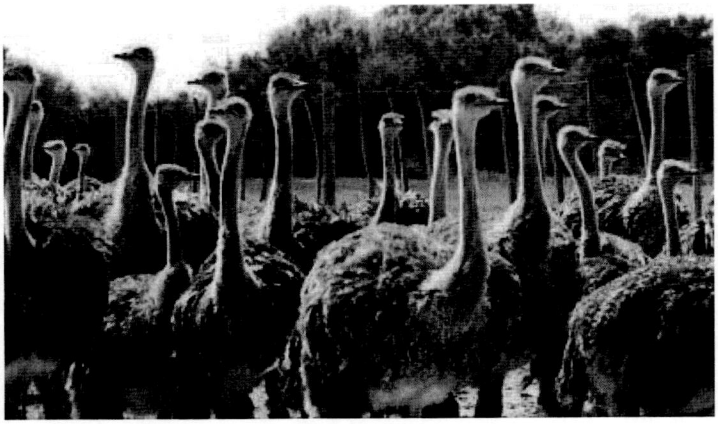

Ostrich Farming

Chapter **6**

Housing of Poultry

Poultry housing is one of the important considerations from long term viability of farming business. The site selection should be appropriate in terms of transport, security, provision of amenities like water, road, electricity, etc. The shelter should provide protection from adverse weather conditions and vectors of diseases like human, rodent and wild birds. The natural light (direct sunlight for at least one-two hours in the day), plenty of oxygen, slow flow of air are essential for good housing.

Site Selection

The following points should be considered for selection of site for establishment of a poultry farm:

a) No Previous Poultry Activity

i) The area should be at a safe distance away from the existing poultry to save birds from any infections.

ii) It should ascertained that no poultry activity is associated with the site previously.

iii) It should be away from where poultry traffic passes.

b) Soil Structure of Land

i) As far as possible harder soil site should be chosen. Black cotton soil increases construction cost.

ii) An elevated area should be preferred.

iii) Drainage should be faster and water accumulation pits should be less. Low lying area will always create problems of flies, mosquitoes and mud.

iv) Land should be even and not rocky.

c) Easy Approach to Farm

i) While planning the poultry business transport facilities should be kept in mind.

A well connected road should be available towards the poultry farm for smooth farm functioning.

d) Water Source is Lifeline

i) Without adequate water resource the existence of farm can not be imagined.

ii) Plenty of water should be available to fulfill the needs of drinking, cleaning of sheds, equipments and for summer cooling.

iii) Quality of water, specially its mineral content and bacterial load should be minimum.

e) Isolation from Human/Animal Accommodation

i) Farm location should be away from human and animal habitations as they act as vectors for many diseases them.

ii) Farm itself may generate obnoxious smell, especially in rainy season.

iii) Animal residence especially dairies may not only create filthy environment and transmit ticks/lice and even increase dangerous gasses levels in the area, hence isolation from them is must.

iv) Less the human/animal movement better for your farm.

f) Availability of electricity

i) Check in advance the availability of 3-phase electric line.

ii) Electricity availability ought to 24 hours or less by 20% but light should be available in night and afternoon.

iii) Less electric light hours means more use of generator set i.e. extra expenditure.

Construction Details of a Poultry House

The roof should be water proof with a proper slope. Generally gable type building is recommended. Shed-type house can be constructed especially if the land available is narrow strip and rainfall expected in the area is scanty. The roof type may be plain concrete laid or made of asbestos sheets in monitor, shed, gable and other forms as shown here.

In case of Brooder-Grower house (BGH), width of the fountain will be more than that of the wall; a monolithic, concrete fountain is preferred.

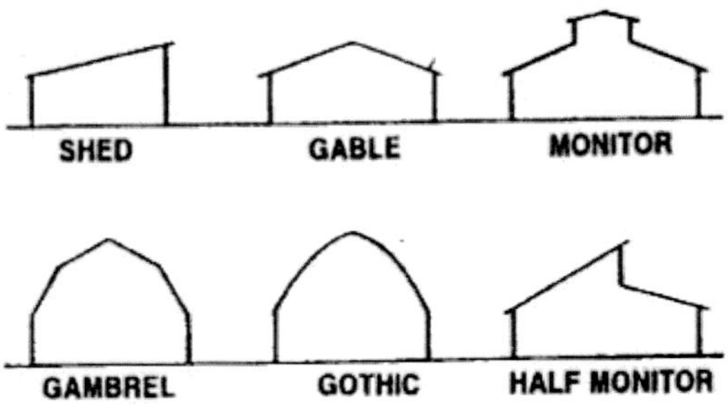

A reinforced cement concrete (RCC) fountain 0.75 to 0.9 m deep and 25-30 cm wide is desirable. BGH is constructed in an elevated area with a plinth of the least 0.60-0.90 m. Full walls can be constructed on either side of long axis, usually made of brick-work with internal finishing by cement plastering and white washed generally side wall should be 2.1-2.4cm (7 to 8ft) to provide slope in the roof on either sides in the areas where temperature is likely to high, the height can be 3.0m (10ft) with height of the building at the centre being 3.6 to 4.2m (12 to 14ft). One-third to one half of the side wall from the floor level is made of brick and the remaining covered by expanded metal. If the climatic conditions are warm throughout the year, the centre side wall, expecting brickwork can be covered with expended metal.

It is common practice to provide door(s) facing East and/or West in gable roof houses and on the side wall with overhang in shed-type houses. The size of a door should be 1.8 m (6ft) high and 1.2 m (4ft) wide.

Normally roof is hoisted on truss-work made of either wood, steel, tiles, red-mud plastic, bitumen sheets, Asbestos, cement concrete sheets or corrugated asbestos sheets or corrugated aluminium sheets. Generally an overhang 0.9 to 1.2m (3 to 4 ft) is provided.

The floor of the Poultry shed should be hygienic, non-porous, easily cleanable, durable, quick-drying, non-slippery, hard warring, non-absorbent of moisture and least expensive. A slope of 1 cm for every 40-60 cm of the solid floor towards the side wall of the house with 5 cm pipes every 3 m (10ft) will help cleaning when the birds are removed.

How to calculate length of the CLH?

The most important factors to be considered are:

1. Cage dimensions
2. Cage arrangement

	W	**D**	**H**
Generally 3 bird laying cages:	45.72 cm (18 inch)	38.10 cm (15 inch)	40.64 cm (16 inch)

with the projection floor by 15.21 cm (6 inch) is used to facilitate rolling of eggs.

The maximum number of tiers of cages is 3. Therefore, 3-tier cage arrangement with 2L and 1M is used in a layer house.

Housing

The following principals for housing and environmental conditions are important for making comfort housing for birds and easy functioning of poultry farming.

a) Physical protection

i) Inside the shed rodent control is a priority consideration. The shed should be rodent proof.

ii) Snakes & reptile may creep inside the shed from rat holes or damaged wire netting.

iii) No open water pits should be left for attracting wild flying birds or wild cats.

b) Floor Space requirement

i) Broiler birds need floor space as per age or targeted body weight to be raised for marketing.

ii) The floor space for Layer chick varies with age. It also varies depending on the type of floor used in the house.

c) Long term investment should be proper

i) Your planning for housing should be on long term basis. Temporary arrangement should be discouraged.

d) Automation saves labour/recurring cost in large farms

i) Automatic or guided drinking water metal/cemented channels will save labour.

ii) Feeding as far as possible should be on conveyor belt type. In small farm automatic out-letting round plastic feeder on deep litter/slat floor is appropriate.

iii) For feeding caged layer moving trolley/belt system may be installed.

Factors Affecting Design of Poultry Houses

Designing of poultry house involves a series of compromise between ideals and feasibility to give best economic performance. Following are the main factors to be considered:

1. Temperature
2. Ventilation
3. Humidity
4. Light
5. Floor, feeder and water space requirements.

1. Temperature

Removal of exercise heat from Poultry houses is the major housing problem in India and other tropical areas. Chicken having a body temperature between 40.5°C to 42.2°C will find it difficult to dissipate much heat through radiation, when atmospheric temperature is above 37°C. Very little heat is lost from the body of birds through evaporative cooling as they do not have sweat glands to perspire. The major mode of dissipating the body heat at high ambient temperature is by panting. Chicken start dying due to heat protraction at 38°C and above. The convention is another mode of heat loss from the birds but the amount of heat loss depends upon the temperature of birds body surface and that of surrounding air, speed or movement of air currents, humidity, etc.

Effect of temperature on laying hen is given in Fig. Although the laying hen, may produce eggs at a maximal rate over the temperature range of 55 to 75°F, the optimal temperature is probably closer to 75°F.

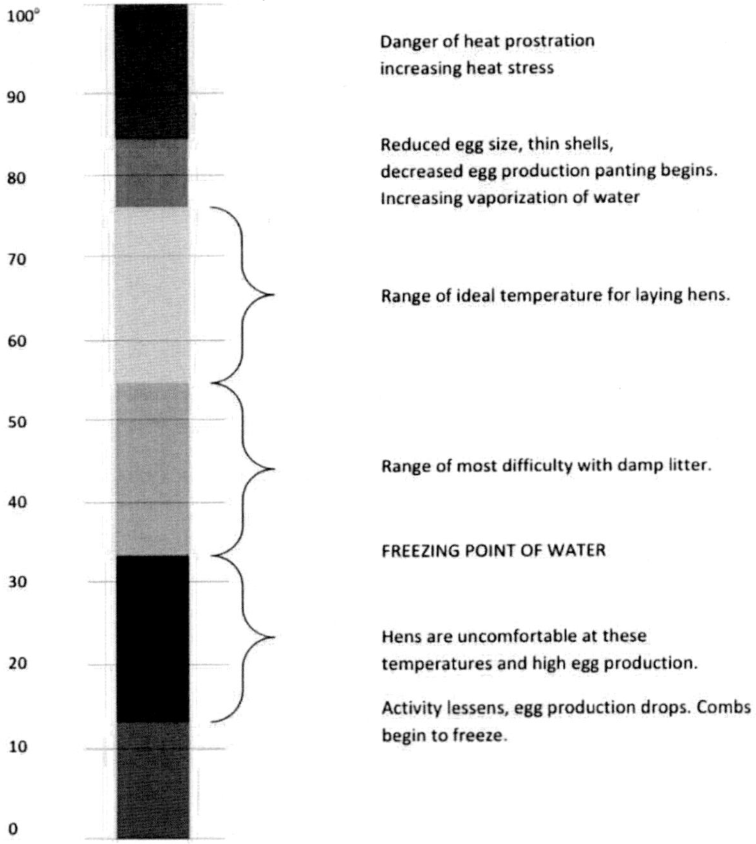

Effect of temperature on the laying hen

2. Ventilation

Proper ventilation requires the movement of fresh air into the building and removal of stale air out of building in such a way to produce a healthy atmosphere in all parts of the house.

Ventilation is required in Poultry house for three reasons:

a) To provide sufficient oxygen for birds to keep them healthy and in peak production. This requirement is easily met and is rearely a limited factor in poultry sheds.

b) To remove ammonia, carbon dioxide, methane and other undesirable gases from poultry sheds. This also includes the removal of moisture given off by birds in their droppings, exhaled gases, spilling from water, etc. to keep the humidity of the atmosphere down to an acceptable level. This is often a limiting factor in most of the poultry houses.

c) To keep the temperature of poultry house down during summer.

A poultry house having height where a poultry attendant can stand in an ordinary condition will have enough air required by birds confined there. However, care should be taken during stress period particularly during heat-stress accompanied with high humidity. Under such circumstances, respiration rate is very high and total volume of air breathed may be eight or ten times more than required.

The amount of air movement needed to keep the litter dry in a poultry house will depend upon the air temperature inside and outside the house and also on humidity gradient inside and outside the house.

Poultry houses in most of the tropical areas are open type with cross ventilation to combat the problems of heat during summer and as a result of this there may be a problem of dry litter rather than wet litter. During rainy season removal of excessive moisture from the poultry shed becomes a problem, when humidity inside and outside are quiter high. Since the houses are open type, there is not much temperature difference also. Under such circumstances, excessive ventilation may not be helpful. Dampness can be reduced only by raising the inside temperature or restricting the movement of air so that inside temperature is raised by itself.

Ventilation is reduced during winter to avoid the loss of heat from the shed but this may lead to dampness and accumulation of ammonia and other stresses. Therefore, it is suggested that ventilation should be maintained high enough to take care of high humidity and other undesirable gases avoiding the direct drought in the shed.

The extent of ventilation in poultry house should compromise between the minimal ventilation required in winter, when it is necessary to conserve all availble heat and maximum requirement of the summer, when it is required to keep the temperatue as low as possible.

3. Humidity

Correct humidity is another important factor for efficient performance of birds in the shed at different stages of life. High humidity in shed is very harmful to birds and it may help development of pathogenic micro-organisms causing diseases in birds. Low humidity in poultry houses results in dry and dusty litter and this might lead to respiratory ailments.

4. Light in Poultry House

The visible light is only part of the radient energy spectrum which falls between 400 to 700 mh. Chicken appear to see better, when the illumination is through long end of the spectrum, otherwise they behave similar to man and have colour vsions.

Light intensity is expressed in "Foot candle"(fc)

The general equation is:

$$\text{Average intensity (fc)} = \frac{\text{Power provided (waltz)}}{\text{Area of surface lit (sq ft)}} \times K$$

Where K is constant of specific light.

Table 1: K-value for light intensity

Colour	Type of lighting	
	Tungsten	Fluorescent
White	5	18
Red	0.3	1.5

There are two factors influencing the intensity of light falling on birds:

1. Power of light source-The amount of light given out by the bulb directly proportional to its wattage.
2. Distance of surface from the light source-the light intensity decreases as the surface of light is placed farther away from the surface.

Housing of Birds

The basic functions of a good poultry house are as follows:

i) Comfortable and relaxing to the broiler/layer bird.

ii) Able to provide sufficient space for feeders and waterers.

iii) Cool in summer and warm in winter & less humidity in rainy seasons.

iv) Protection against direct sunlight, rain and wind.

v) Always should be dry with least dampness.

vi) Sensible air circulation.

vii) Rodent, wild flying bird and local birds should have no excess inside shed.

The following housing systems may be adopted for rearing of poultry:

A. Deep Litter House

The other features of deep litter house are as follows:

i) The side walls north-west direction are open and covered with wire netting to the height of 6-9 feet above the ground level. The ground level should be 1.5 - 2.0 feet above the ground to protect from entry of rain water.

ii) The width of shed ~~is~~ should be usually less than 30 feet.

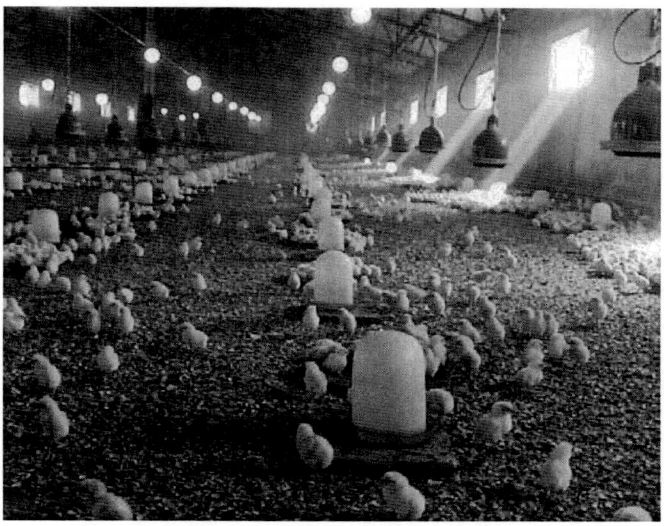

Deep litter system of housing

iii) Length of the building depends on number of birds to be housed. Length should not exceed 4 to 6 times the width.

iv) The side walls should be 2-3 feet high and above it wire net should be fixed.

v) The floor should be cement concrete.

vi) The roof should be of asbestos sheets supported by iron pipes/ angles.

vii) Deep litter system is used for housing layer flocks (from day old age to 72 weeks of age) and broilers both.

viii) On the floor litter is spread initially 1½ - 2 inches thick and with advancement of time it is supplemented till its thickness reaches 6-9 inches in depth by fresh litter material. Commonly used litter materials are rise-husk, wood-shavings and saw dust.

ix) The floor space needed per bird varies with the age and size of birds.

Table 2: The floor space requirement under deep litter system

Age group (weeks)	Floor space requirement sq.ft./chick
0-4	0.5
8	1
16	1.5
16-20	2
20-72	2.5

In shed where automatic feeder and waterer are used, the space requirement per bird declines proportionately.

x) The deep litter absorbs dropping moisture and reduces its weight. A layer hybrid voids about 60-75 kg. Wet faeces which contains about 85% moisture producing 12-15 kg dry matter. A broiler voids about 0.75 - 1.25 kg dried faecal material in 5 weeks period.

B. Slat Housing

This housing system is an improved modified method over that of deep litter system. Here, a portion of the deep litter shed is raised above the ground and welded metal / wooden pieces are fixed. Other features of slat system of housing are:

i) Commonly 40-60 per cent area of shed is converted as slatted floor.

ii) Wooden pieces of 1- 1¼ inch width x 1" thick and about 6 ft. long pieces are fixed at a distance of 1-1¼ inches on a base giving it a shape of channel.

iii) The slat of 1" x 1" wire welded mesh of 10 gauge thickness can be used to form slatted floor.

iv) The area of slatted floor is made in the middle of shed length leaving space for deep litter at all the four sides. The slatted floor can also be prepared close to one wall. The side wall height of deep litter house should be 2-3 ft.

v) Below the slatted floor the covered area is for faecal collection. The birds prefer to rest on slatted floor.

vi) Waterer/water channel are usually located on slatted area.

The slatted floor can be used for rearing commercial broiler and layer flock and it can accommodate 25-30 per cent more birds than the simple deep litter shed. As maximum faecal dropping is collected inside slatted floor, the deep litter area remains less dirty.

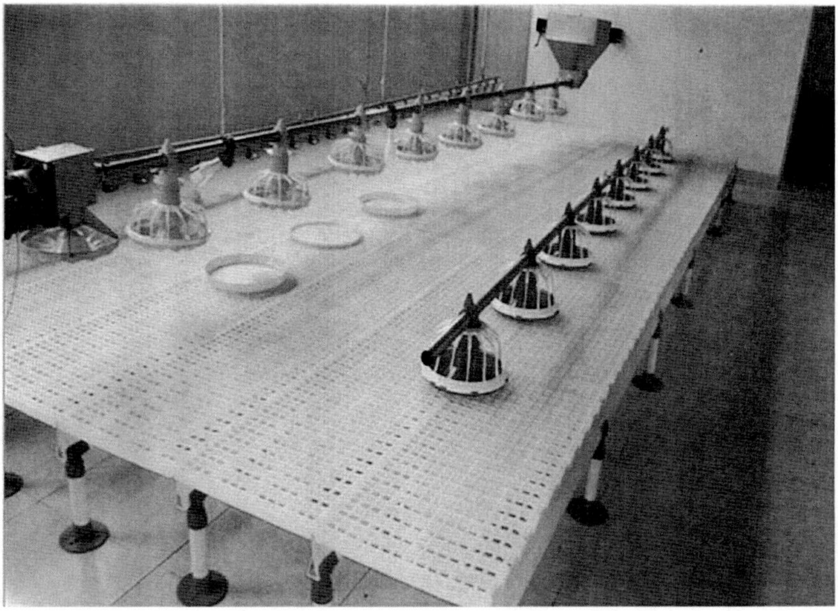

Slat system of housing

Cage Housing

The salient features of cage housing are as follows:

a) Raised platform layer cage house

The modernization and force to make poultry keep an economically viable enterprise, the old methods of keeping birds have dramatically changed in last 50 years. Now-a-days raised platform layer cage house is very popular which has following features:

i) The platform to fix cages is raised 6-10 feet above ground level on all sides.

ii) Raised platform keeps away the birds from obnoxious gases, makes it easy to remove collected faecal matter mechanically, and due to free movement of air oxygen and carbon dioxide levels remains optimum.

b) Cages for broiler rearing

In India, method of rearing broiler in cages is less prevalent but in developed countries it is a normal practice. The salient points of cages are as follows :

i) The cages with the size of 1½ x 4 x 1½ (width, length, height) ft^3 are arranged in a row in open side sheds in single or two tiers. Each compartment house may accommodate 15-20 broilers and 25-30 layer chicks.

ii) Chicks are placed on day old age and remain in cage till age of disposal. Automatic watering system and feeder belt system/ manual is arranged as per the size of operation.

iii) In developed countries removable welded wire or plastic coated coup cages of 18 x 18 x 48 $inches^3$ to accommodate 20 broilers (1.5 kg each) are used. These are fitted with automatic waterer and feeder.

c) Cages for egg production

It is well known that the revolution in egg production is due to cage rearing. In a smaller place by providing 60-66 square inches of space per bird in 3 tiers enormously increase the utility of space. Cages can be used for chicks, growers and layer independently or jointly. Let us examine housing need for each category.

1. Chick raising cages

i) Day old chicks can be raised up to 6 weeks of age on wire cages.

ii) Usually cages are of size 48" x 36" x 12". In each cage, 31-40 chicks are placed or 20-40 sq. inch space is given per bird.

iii) To provide heat a bulb of 60-100 watt is placed hanging from top inside the cage or complete house is heated.

iv) These cages can be placed as 2 or 3 tiers electricity problem exists.

2. Grower Raising Cages

You can house growers in specially designed grower-cages. Few salient points are as follows:

i) Normal size of grower compartment is 1½ x 3 square feet for 18 pullets.

ii) These are like layer cages with two exceptions i.e. the cage floor welded wire mesh in 1" x 1" in place of 1" x 3". Secondly are devoid of egg-slant in front for rolling out the egg out side the sitting area.

iii) Cages can be fixed in 2-3 tiers.

3. Layer Raising Cage

In a shed pullets are usually housed in groups of three in 16" x 12" x 18" sized compartment. Each bird receives 60-66 sq. inches space for housing.

i) Each adult female is provided with 3" length feeder space across cage length and 2" running length running waterer space in galvanized channel.

ii) Layer cages in open shed system are organized in 3 tiers, however, in automatic controlled shed may accommodate 6-8 tiers as per facilities.

iii) Cage floor welded wire mesh size is 1" x 3", whereas other side could be 2" x 4" or 3" x 4" size depends as per bird's size at the time of housing which reduce cost also.

iv) Cage housing increased the density at least three times to that of deep litter but have easier management of flock and minimize labour cost.

v) Availability of feed, water and space need for comfortable housing are fulfilled leading for cleaner eggs and minimum feeder wastage.

Different cages sizes depending upon the capacity of birds

45 x 30 cm for 3 birds

45 x 40 cm for 4 birds

50 x 35 cm for 4 birds

50 x 45 cm for 5 birds

60 x 37.5 cm for 5 birds

According to the number of birds in a cage, it may be categorized into:

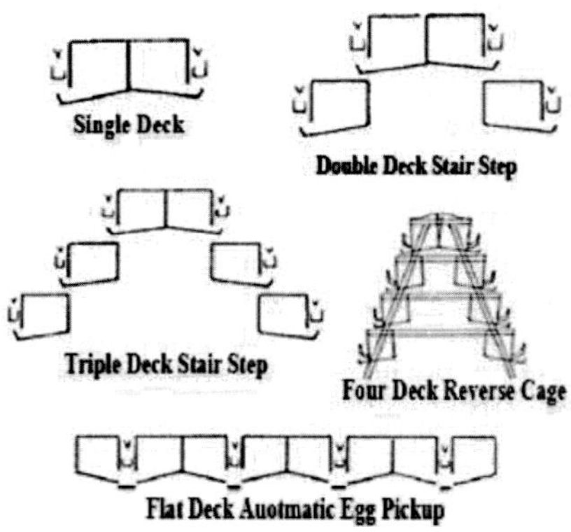

1. Single-bird Cages : The first laying cages were suited to one bird but as the investment is high, single bird cages are seldom used today.
2. Multiple-bird Cages : These laying cages hold two or more birds, but usually not more than eight or ten, with three or four being the most common.
3. Colony Cages : These are large laying cages suitable for holding between 20 and 30 pullets. To conserve space, thereby reducing the investment in the house in which the laying cages are placed. At present the following general classification of cage arrangement are available:
   - Single-Deck : It involves placing one tier of cages in a house. In this cage arrangement, there is high investment.
   - Double-Deck : These are popular because the upper deck is offset, allowing the dropping to fall through the wise mesh to the house floor without touching the lower deck. The offset arrangement is often called the stair-step system.
   - Triple-Deck : To conserve house space still, further, three decks are common.

- Four-Deck : Same as triple-deck except that four decks are used.
- Five-Deck: Same as triple-deck except that five decks are sued.
- Flat-Deck : Although these are single-deck cage installations the cages areplaced close together without walk way for servicing the pullets. All such work is done from a motorised catwalk.

Modern Poultry Housing

The genetic potential of poultry cannot be fully exploited unless they are given the comfortable environment in the house. The proper environment has an impact on health and well-being of the birds. Thus, the modern housing known as "Environment Controlled (EC) house is in vogue.

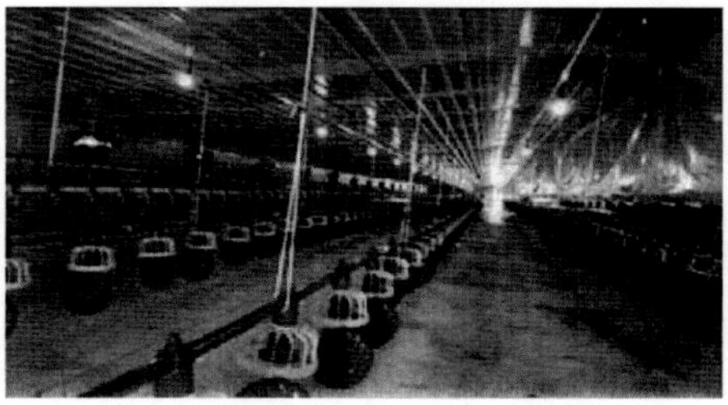

EC house

Optimum environmental conditions must be provided for the maximum genetic potential and fed conversion ratio of birds. The heat production through digestion and metabolism should be equal to the heat lost by the bird through conduction, convection, radiation and evaporation to maintain their thermal balance. The temperature at which the birds achieve the thermal balance is called Critical temperature. The laying hens perform with little or no discomfort within a temperature range of 50-77^{0}F (10-24^{0}C). It is called the comfort zone. Additional nutrients are required to produce heat to keep the body warm at the temperature below the comfort zone. Also, more nutrients are needed to keep the body cool through panting, when temperature is above the comfort zone. The temperature range in which the birds have maximum egg production and feed efficiency is called the optimum temperature. This range is 55-70^{0}F (13-21^{0}C) for layer. The critical temperature and comfort zones vary with different species, age, breed and physiological and productive status. The variation with age is large in chicken. The comfort zone for body chicks is 92-95^{0}F (33-35^{0}C), whereas for adult layers it is 50 to 75^{0}F (10-24^{0}C).

Environmentally controlled poultry housed are designed to operate such that the environmental conditions of temperature, relative humidity, ammonia, carbon dioxide, wind velocity, light, etc. are automatically maintained as near as possible to the optimum range required by the birds.

The sheds constructed are windowless, completely enclosed and insulted. Air is removed from the house through exhaust fan and fresh air is pumped in through intake openings. Natural daylight is not available as the house is illuminated using artificial light. In extreme hot conditions, inside temperature control devices are used. The house does not require any heating except during brooding. The heat produced by the birds is used to maintain inside temperature within the comfortable range for the birds. The ideal environmental conditions maintained in these housed and insulation of ceiling and walls of the house are as follows:

- Temperature 13-21^{0}C
- Humidity 50.75
- Ventilation rate 2-4cfm
- Light 1.0 foot candle for 16 hours
- Moisture content of litter 40%

The structural insulation of ceiling and walls of the house are similar except that it has a gable roof and insulation of both sides and top. The overhang of the roof is reduced to 0.25 m. The width of the house can be increased upto 50ft (15.5m) as the air is mechanically exhausted. Mechanical air movement through the environmentally controlled house is a must to supply oxygen and to remove moisture, ammonia and carbon dioxide and maintain optimum temperature. Typical ventilation fans of 30 inch (0.0m) to 54 in (1.4m) diameter are used for ventilation depending upon the size of the house. The ventilation system in environmentally controlled house must ensure that the air movement in the house is uniform from top to bottom and from side to side. In modern environmentally controlled house, all the environmental requirements are controlled through various computerised sensing devices and operate automatically. These housed are most common in those regions, where power supply is not a problem.

Advantages

- Birds are comfortable and remain healthy.
- Feed efficiency is better.
- Growth/egg production is higher.
- Feeding, watering, egg collection, egg grading and egg packing are controlled automatically and thus, save labour cost.
- More birds can be kept per unit of land area.
- There is no seasonal influence in the performance of birds.

Disadvantages

- Initial cost is high
- Uninterrupted power supply is needed
- Huge losses may occur in case of power failures.

❑❑❑

Chapter 7

Poultry Farm Equipments

In our day-to-day routine activities, we use many appliances/ equipment and utensils for our wellbeing. Similarly, in a Poultry farm, it is essential to use a number of appliances/equipment and utensils in order to keep the birds comfortable and to perform the routine management. Use of equipment in a poultry farm will help in:

- Saving time, labour and cost
- Help in easy functioning of the farm
- Providing comfort to the birds
- Maintaining the health of the birds

Care and Maintenance of Equipment / Utensils

Care and maintenance of equipment and utensils in proper condition is essential for the safety of the birds and longevity of the equipment and utensils. For effective utilization of these equipment and utensils, the following should be practised:

- Only the required number of equipment/utensil should be used in the shed.
- All the equipment and utensil should be thoroughly cleaned, disinfected and dried before use.
- Equipment and utensil should be cleaned regularly.
- Do not shift or use the equipment and utensil from one shed to another without cleaning and disinfection, as they may act as a source of spreading of disease.
- Do not use broken or defective equipment/utensil, as they may harm birds.
- Immediately remove/dispose and replace broken or defective equipment/utensil.

- After use, equipment especially those with sharp edges should be kept in a safe place out of reach of the birds.
- Electrical equipment like debeaker should always be kept in working condition.
- Fragile equipment/utensils like egg filler flats should be handled gently and carefully to avoid breakage.
- Equipment/utensil made of iron like feeder should be kept dry to avoid rusting.

Different types of equipment

Different type of equipments and utensils are required for different activities and for different age groups. For example, brooder is used only for chicks and helps in providing heat to the chicks in order to keep them comfortable. Therefore, it is important to learn about the different equipment and utensils required in broiler and layer farms. Thorough knowledge on the poultry farm equipment will also help in understanding the quantity required, their placement and uses of each one of them. In this lesson, your will be introduced to different farm equipment, which are commonly used in a poultry farm.

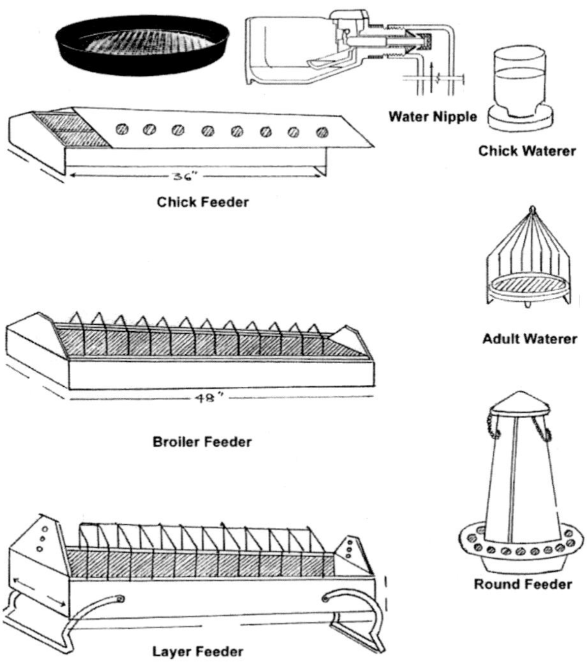

Common Equipment used in a poultry farm

- Identify different equipment and utensils used in a poultry farm;
- Explain their characteristics and uses in routine farm activities;
- Care and maintain these equipment and utensils.

Equipment used in a poultry farm

In India, generally, broilers are reared on the floor (deep litter system) and layers in cages. Therefore, the requirement of some of the equipment in broiler farm varies from that of layer farm. In this section, you will learn about the different equipment used in a broiler and layer farm.

Broiler farm equipments

Different equipment used in a broiler farm are as follows:

i) **Brooders :** The newly hatched chicks' body temperature regulatory system is not well-developed and hence, they should be provided warmth especially during the first 3 to 4 weeks of age. Under natural conditions, hen provides warmth to the chicks. Whereas, in a poultry farm, brooder acts like an artificial hen and provide heat/ warmth to the chicks and also acts as a source of light. A brooder consists of a heating source, reflectors to reflect the heat and light towards the ground and other accessories like stand, light and heat adjusting devices (thermostats), etc. There are different types of brooders available in the market and the details are discussed below:

- **Canopy Brooder :** It is an inverted umbrella-like ("canopy" shaped) equipment made up of Galvanized Iron (GI) or bamboo basket (2 to 3 feet in diameter) with 3 electric bulb points.

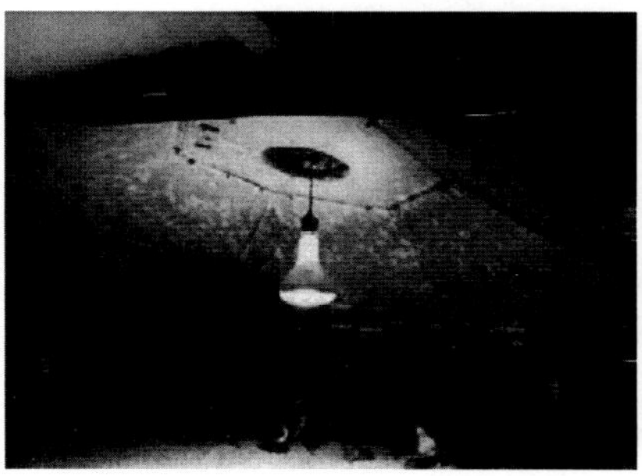
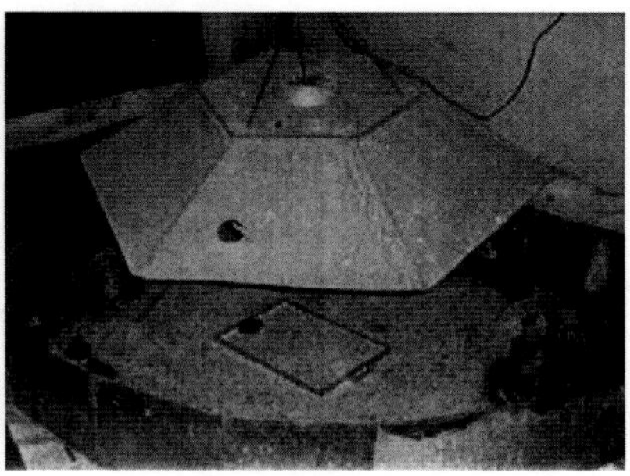

Canopy Brooders

- **Reflector Brooder :** This electrical brooder consists of a rectangular shaped reflecting surface, with a bulb point to fix an electric bulb and a thermostat for regulating temperature. Though they are durable and reliable, they are expensive.
- **Infra-red Bulb Brooder :** This type of brooder uses infra-red bulb as heating source. The infra-red bulbs with 150 and 250 Watts capacities are available in the market.

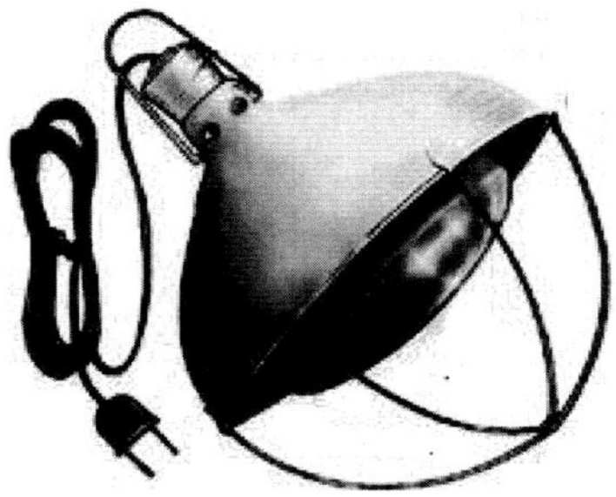

Infra-red bulb brooder

- **Battery Brooder :** As the name suggests, a battery brooder consists of 3 to 4 tiers (rows) of batteries (brooding space). Each tier consists of a 'heating space' and a 'run space'. Heating space which accounts to one-third (33%) of the total space consists of a reflector brooder. Run space which occupies two-third (67%) of the total space is used for feeding, watering and movement of birds. Generally, they are used for brooding Japanese quails.

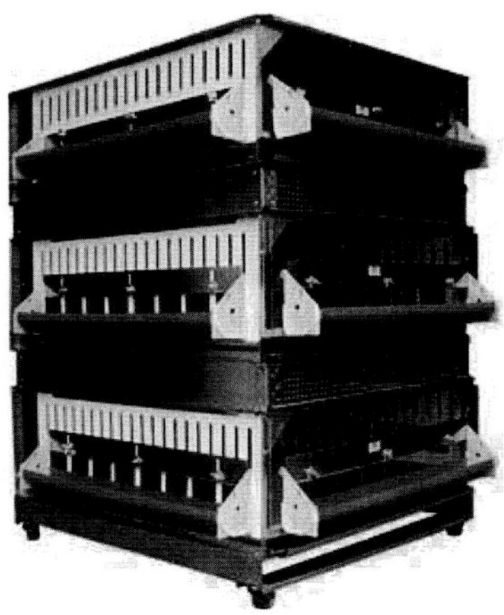

Battery Brooder

A farmer can choose any one of the brooders mentioned above as per the requirements and availability. Thumb rule is that one brooder is required for every 200 to 250 chicks initially, depending on the local environmental conditions.

ii) **Brooder Guard :** The brooder or chick guard is used to restrict the movement of chicks to keep close to the brooders and feed and water source as they are very active, roam aimlessly and may move away from the heat source, feed and water. Generally, brooder guard is a circular arrangement made up of a number of rectangular structure (wire mesh or thin sheets of metal or cardboard or bamboo mat) each measuring about 2 ft x 1 ft linked by hooks. However, varying heights and lengths are available in the market depending upon the requirement and age of the birds. As the chick grows, the area provided to the chicks within the brooder guard also changes accordingly.

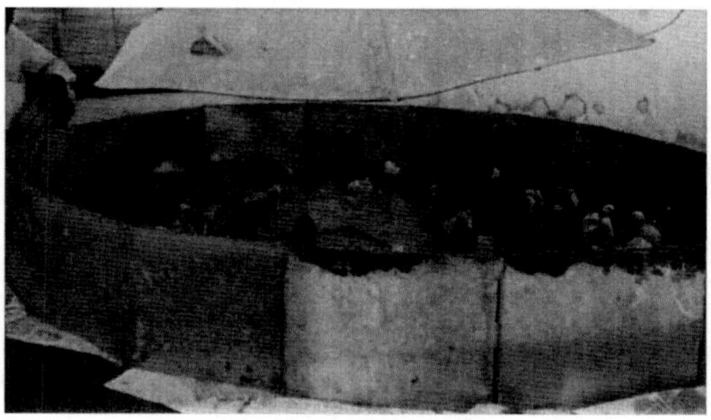

Brooder Guard

iii) **Feeders :** Feeders are equipment used for feeding the birds. They may be conventional or semi-automatic and are available in various designs and shapes. Feeders are used both in the brooder house and broiler house. Chick feeder normally are 3-5 feet in length and 1½" - 2" in depth fitted with strong wire pieces to prevent entry of chicks inside the feeder. Two types of feeders are used for broilers *viz.* linear (long) feeders made of iron and circular feeders made of high-impact plastic. For raising large number of chicks in a commercial broiler farm, automatic feeding system can be fitted having feed trough, chain with pulley, tube and conveyed belt.

- **Linear feeders :** They are straight, wedge-shaped, placed on the floor and usually made of Galvanised Iron (GI) or locally available materials like wood, bamboo, etc. One of the major advantages of linear feeder is that birds can feed on either side of the feeder and hence, total feeding space available will be two times the length of the feeder. However, the main disadvantage with the linear feeder is that birds may try to enter into the feeder and search for grains or may topple them resulting in wastage of feed. Therefore, grills are provided to prevent the entry of birds into the feeder. In addition, linear feeders need to be filled to ½ or 1 level every day. The dimensions of linear chick feeder and linear broiler feeder are tabulated below:

Table 1: Dimensions of feeders for broiler chicken

Feeder	Length (cm)	Width (cm)	Height (cm)	Grill Space
Linear chick feeders	60 to 75	7.5 at the base and 10 the top	5	2.5 cm apart
Linear grower feeders	90 to 150	15 at the base and 25 the top	7.5 to 10	5 cm apart

In both type of feeders, grill can be easily opened for filling of feed and adjustable stands are fixed to the base at suitable intervals to facilitate raising of the level at which feed is available for the broilers.

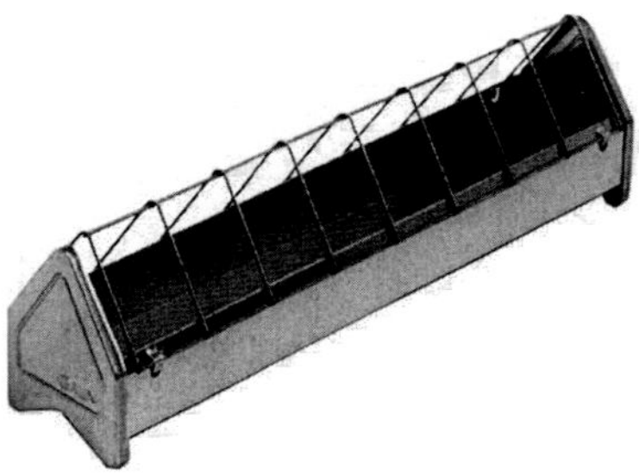

Linear feeder with grill

- **Circular feeders :** They are circle-shaped and usually made of strong plastic. They are also called "hanging feeders" because they are usually suspended (hanged) from the roof or pipeline and never kept on the floor. Circular feeders have a base plate and a bell portion. Since they are hanging and feed is supplied through pipeline, as and when feed is consumed by the chicks, the feed freely flows from the bell on to the base plate and hence, feed is available all the time. The major advantages of circular feeder are its easy maintenance, feed is available round the clock and 30% more birds can stand and eat when compared to linear feeders. They are available in different sizes and usually bright coloured (red or blue) to attract broilers, especially chicks to the feed. When completely full, depending on age and number of birds feeding on them, the feed will be sufficient for 4 to 7 days.

The feed should be available at the level of the back of birds in order to minimize feed spillage. At the beginning of brooding, the base plate should be about 5 to 6 cm (2 to 2½ inches) above the floor and should be increased as the birds grow. For adjusting the height of the feeder, simple clamps are provided in the feeder.

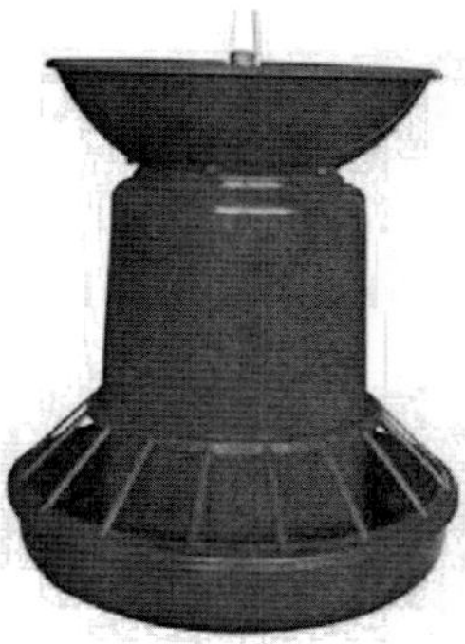

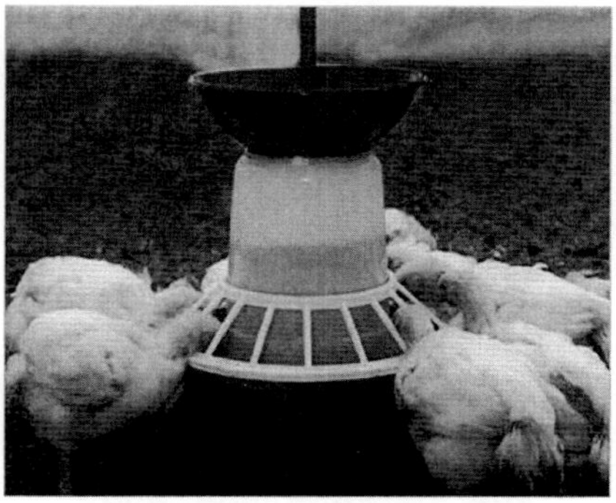

Circular feeder

- **Type of feeder to be used :** Since both the types of feeders are having their own advantages and disadvantages, a farmer can choose any one type of feeder depending upon the requirement and availability.
- **Number of feeders required :** The number of feeders required depends on the type of feeder used (linear or circular) and the age of the birds. In case of linear feeder, about 30 broilers up to 4 weeks of age can eat in one linear feeder. One circular feeder is sufficient for 28 chicks and therefore 36 feeders are required for 1,000 chicks. Similarly, for broiler birds at market, one circular feeder is sufficient for 19 birds and therefore, 54 feeders are required for 1,000 birds.

iv) **Drinkers or waterer :** Drinkers are the equipments used for providing water to the chicks and birds. They are of two types *viz.* linear and circular. However, circular drinkers are more commonly used than linear drinkers. Linear drinkers are placed on the floor and circular drinkers ("Hanging drinkers") are hung from the top and are connected to an overhead tank. Similar to feeders, circular drinkers should be kept at an appropriate height so that water is available at the level of back of the birds. There are different types of circular drinkers available in the market.

- **Fountain drinker :** They are manual drinkers used for chicks during first week of brooding and are kept on the floor. One of the main advantages of fountain drinker is that when a chick or bird drinks water, it automatically comes out of the holes similar to the fountain and hence the named "fountain drinker". It is also easy to give vitamins, medicines or vaccines through this drinker. One fountain drinker is sufficient for 100 chicks and therefore, for 1,000 birds, 10 foundation drinkers are required.

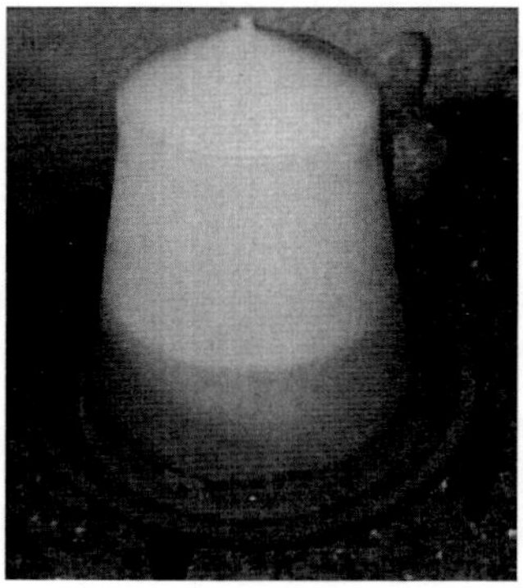

Fountain drinker

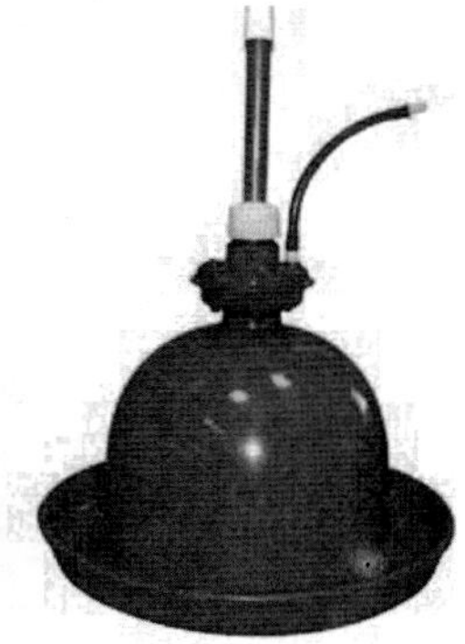

Bell drinker

- **Bell drinker :** They are bell-shaped, bright coloured (red or blue), made up of high-impact plastic and used after one to two weeks of age. They are hung from the top and never kept on the floor: Similar to the feeders, height of the drinker can be adjusted using simple clamp mechanism and the rate of flow of water is adjustable by a valve. One bell drinker is sufficient for 94 broiler chicks and therefore for 1,000 birds, 11 bell drinkers are required. Similarly, one bell drinker is sufficient for 57 broiler birds, and therefore, 18 bell drinkers are required for 1,000 birds.

For selecting the type of drinker to be used in a broiler farm, there is no hard and fast rules and hence a farmer can choose any type of drinker depending upon the requirement and availability.

Layer farm equipments

In the previous chapter, it has already been discussed that a layer farm has two types of houses *viz.* brood-grow houses (BGH) and layer house or cage layer houses (CLH). Different equipment are required in each of the houses.

a) In Brood-Grow House

The equipments required are same as discussed in a broiler house. However, the requirement of feeder and drinker space are different and therefore, only the number of each of them required changes.

i) **Brooders :** Same as discussed under broilers

ii) **Brooder Guard :** Same as discussed under broilers

iii) **Chick Feeders :** Same as discussed under broilers. Each hanging feeder is sufficient for about 28 birds and therefore, about 36 feeders are needed for 1,000 birds.

iv) **Grower Feeders :** These are similar to hanging feeders for broilers but are of larger diameter.

v) **Drinkers :** Each bell-drinkers is be sufficient for about 62 chicks and for 1,000 chicks about 20 drinkers are needed.

b) In Layer House

Layers can be reared on deep litter system or cage system. Cage system of rearing is more popular for layers than deep litter system. The equipment used varies depending on the system of rearing. For example, in deep litter system, feeders, drinkers and nest boxes are required. Whereas, in cage system, the cage itself contains drinker, feeder and egg collecting space/tray.

The different equipment required in a layer house covering both the systems:

i) **Feeder :** If the layers are reared on deep litter system, individual plastic round layer feeder storing 7-10 kg feed is hanged in a row. One feeder is sufficient for 30-40 layers depending on weight/size of bird.

ii) **Drinker :** Bell drinker as discussed in broiler house is used.

iii) **Cages :** Layers are generally housed in cages. The most commonly used are 3-bird laying cages as compared to 1, 2, 4, 15 or 30-bird cages. A 3-bird laying cages measures 45 cm (18 inches) in width, 38 cm (15 inches) in depth and 40 cm (16 inches) in height. Each cage has provisions for the birds to eat (feeding channel), drink (Nipple drinker) and egg collection. The maximum number of tiers of cages generally adopted is 3. Therefore, 3- tier cage can be arranged in the shape of 2 L and 1 M.

- **Feeding Channel :** Long aluminum/galvanized sheet feeding channel are fitted in the front side of the cage which runs along the width of the cage and 15 cm (6 inches) above the egg collection channel. The birds consume feed by bringing their heads out through the mesh in front from the feeding channel.
- **Drinkers or Watering Channel :** Aluminum water channel can be fitted with fixed 7.5 to 10.0 cm above the feeding channel. However, such water channels are not preferred due to many disadvantages like requirement of daily cleaning of the channel, overflowing of water leading to high humidity, fly and odour problems as well as occasional empty channels leading to thirst and reduced performance. To overcome these problems, nipples drinkers are used nowadays in the cages.

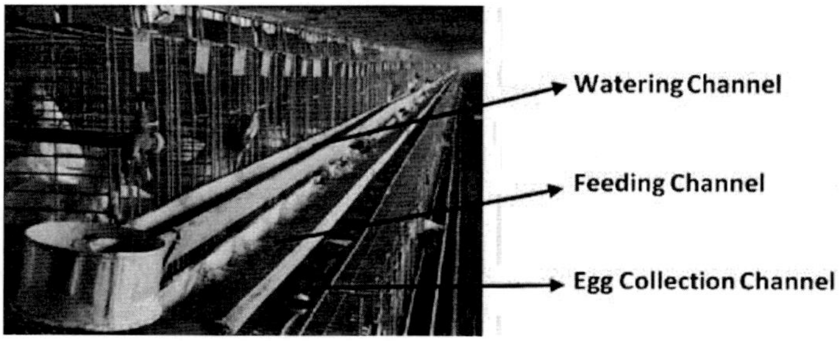

Cage with feeding, watering and egg collection channels

- **Nipple drinkers :** This type of drinkers which is fitted inside the cages at the top edge in the front end of the cage look like a nipple and therefore, it is called "nipple drinker". When a bird presses the nipple with its beak, water automatically comes out. Though they can be used for any type of housing system; they are most commonly used in cages. They are fitted inside the laying cage at 5 cm above the head of the birds so that they can easily hit at the nipple. One nipple drinker in each cage housing 3 layers is sufficient.

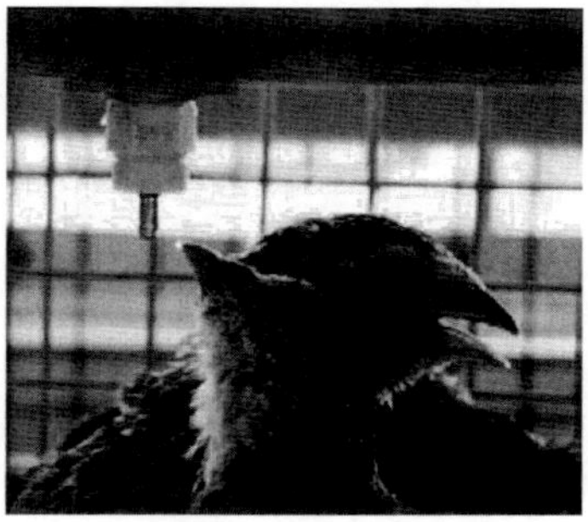

Nipple drinker

- **Egg Collection Channel :** For collection of eggs, the floor of the cage projects by 15 cm (6 inches) with a gradual slope for easy rolling of eggs.

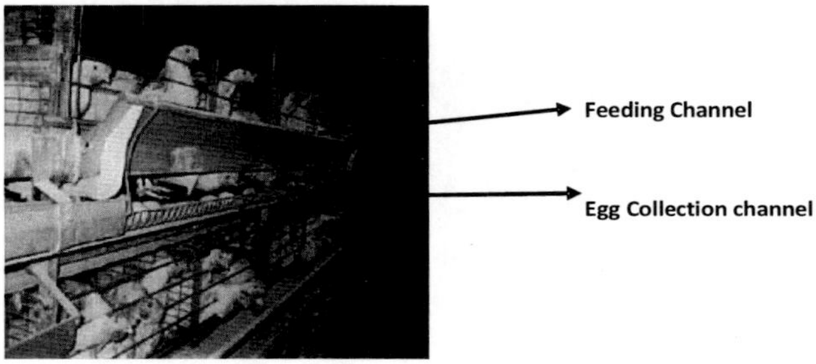

Cage with Egg Collection Channel

v) **Egg Filler Flats :** They are rectangular trays with depressions to hold eggs. They are made of plastic or paper pulp and can hold 30 eggs. Plastic ones are common because they are durable and easy to clean and maintain. However, paper pulp trays reduce breakage of eggs during transportation and are environment-friendly. Eggs are directly collected and transported in egg filler flats.

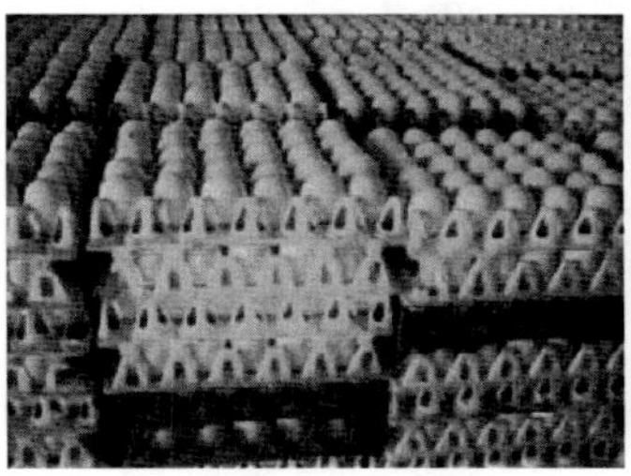

Plastic Egg Filler flats

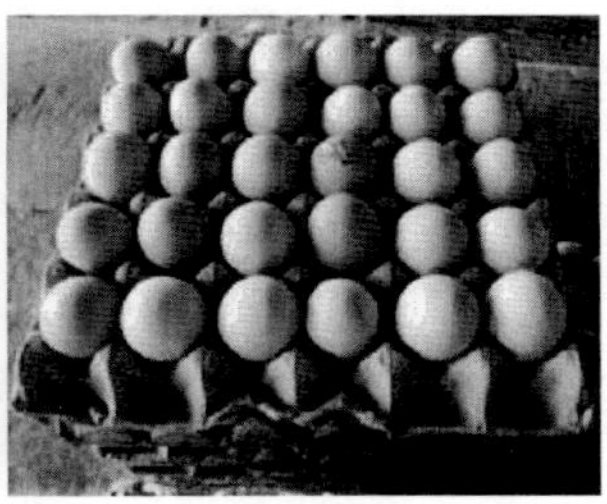

Paper pulp Egg Filler flats

vi) **Nest box :** Nests are not required, when the layers are grown in cages. However, if layers are grown on deep litter system, nests at the rate of 30 per 100 layers have to be provided. In order to get clean and undamaged eggs and to avoid floor eggs, they are constructed or placed inside the shed for laying hens. The sitting place should be isolated, slightly of less light, with soft bedding. Open next box and colony nest boxes made of iron shed with roll-out egg system are preferred. The colony box of size 2' wide and 4-6 ft in length with partition at 12x 14" distance inside are generally recommended. Nests should have an inclined roof because layers have a tendency to jump/fly (Perch) and sit on the nests and may lay eggs.

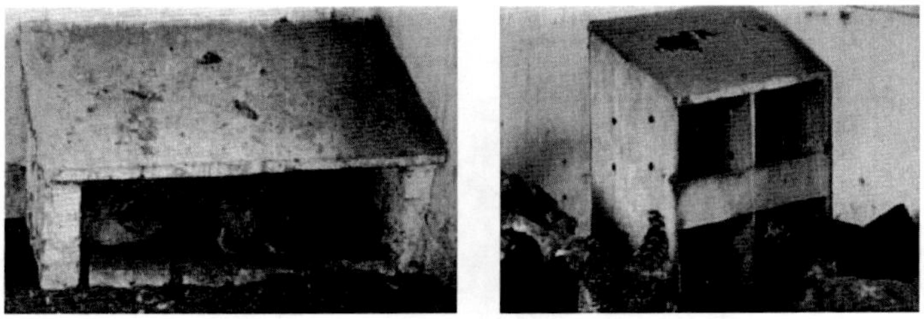

Nest Box

vii) **Candler :** It is electric equipment which produces a beam of light when passed through an egg in dark environment and helps to get an idea about the internal quality of eggs. It is a simple technique used to easily identify cracks in the shell and other defects inside the egg without breaking open the egg. Candling of eggs helps to remove/eliminate cracked eggs or eggs with foreign matter inside like blood spots, meat spots, etc. and used in the grading and sorting of eggs.

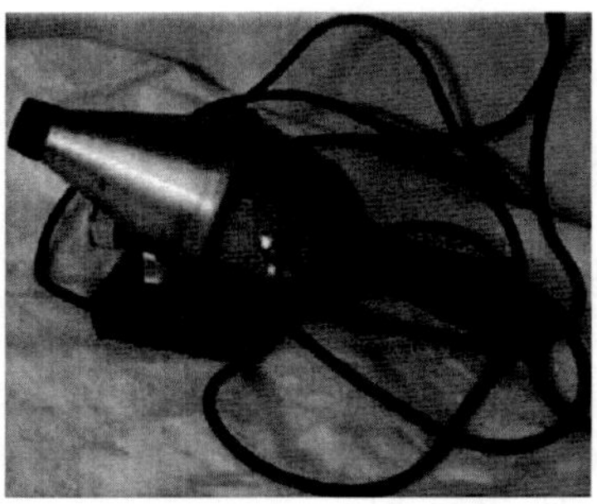

Candler

Other Equipment Used in Poultry Farm

In addition to the equipment described above, for routine farm activities, the following equipment are required:

i) **Automatic Vaccinator :** It is used during vaccination for injecting different doses of vaccine to a large number of birds within short period.

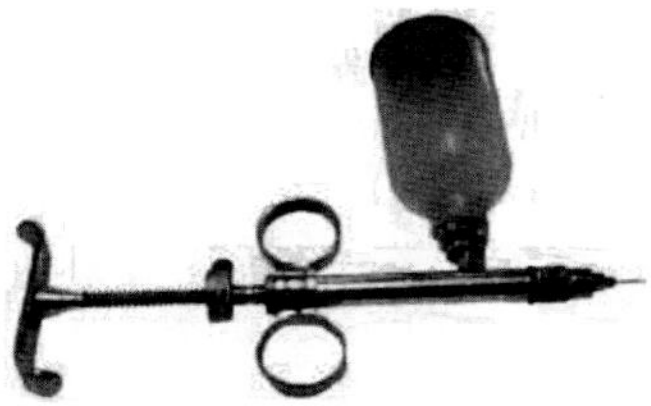

Automatic Vaccinator

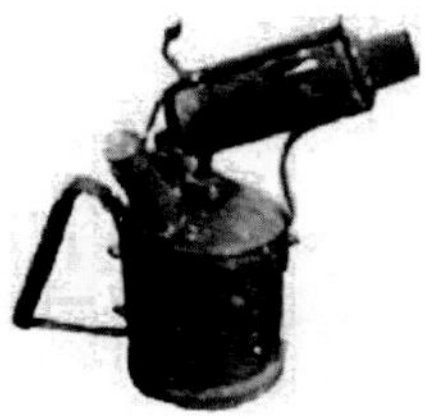

Blow lamp

ii) **Blow-lamp :** Blow-lamp also known as flaming gun is used for disinfection and control of parasites. Usually, kerosene or gas is used in blow-lamp. It is used to flame metal frames or on GI. In either case, after cleaning and disinfection, blow-lamp can be used on the area.

iii) **Buckets :** They are vessels made up of plastic or metal used for carrying feed/water and other materials from one place to another.

iv) **Catching mesh and catching hook:** They are used in broiler farms in order to catch the birds for shifting or routine examination or administration of medicines. Catching mesh consists of several pieces of meshwork (2.5 cm x 2.5 cm or 7.5 cm x 7.5 cm) measuring 60 cm x 60 cm beaded on all sides to protect from sharp edges. These pieces (about 8 to 10 in number) are linked through rings, so that they can be folded and spread whenever needed. When birds need to be caught, they are moved to a corner of the shed, and the catching mesh is spread leaving as much space as possible all round so that the birds cannot escape. Catching hook is a hook with a long handle which can be used to catch the birds by the leg.

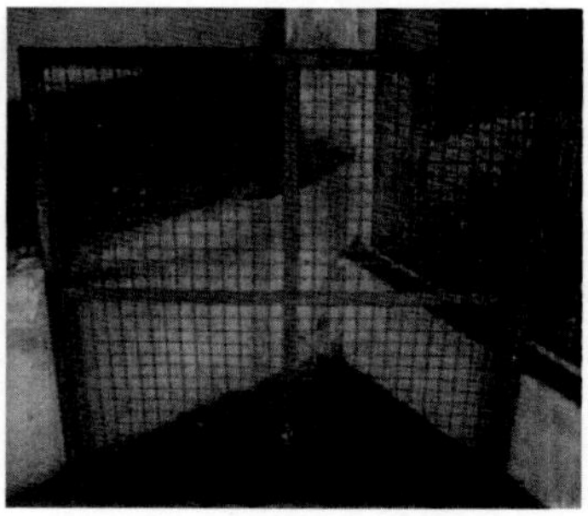

Unit of catching mesh

v) **Crates (Transportation cages) :** Crates are box-like structures made of meshwork or plastic used for transportation of birds. Plastic crates are preferred due to their light weight, durability and easy to handle and clean. The bottom of the crates should be made of meshwork (2.5 cm x 2.5 cm) so that the birds are comfortable in it. All sides are of meshwork 7.5 cm x 7.5 cm so that good ventilation is possible. For loading and unloading, an opening with a lid is provided on the top of the crate. A crate of dimensions 90 cm x 45 cm and of height 30 cm can easily accommodate 10 to 15 broilers depending on body weight.

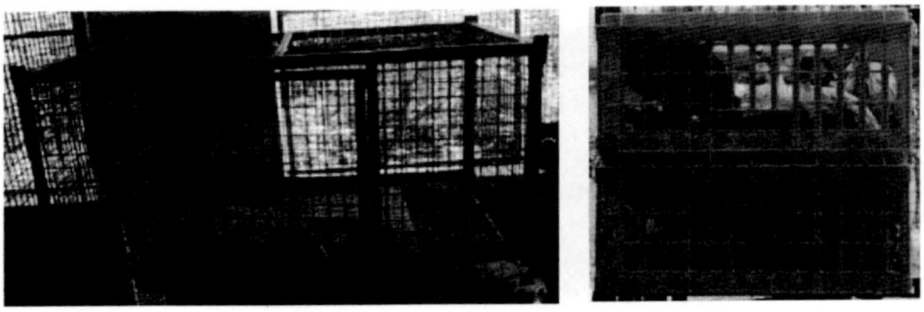

Crates

vi) **Curtains :** Curtains are used to prevent entry of cold wind into the poultry shed during winter conditions. This is particularly necessary during the first 2 to 3 weeks of age when the chicks cannot maintain their body temperature efficiently. Arrangement to close the sidewalls and open in part or full by rolling down, as the day progresses is also necessary.

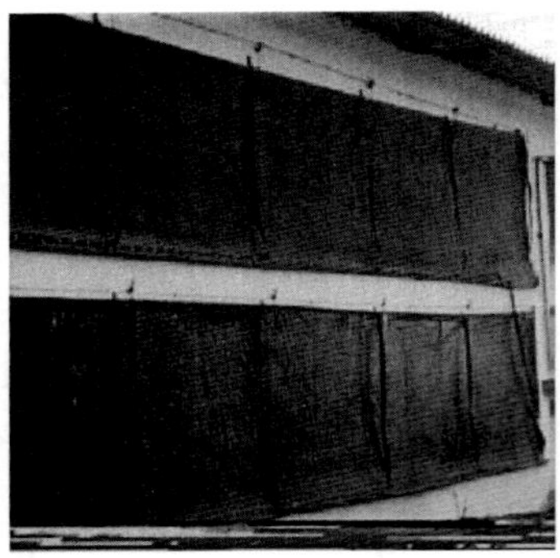

Curtains

vii) **Debeaker :** Debeaker is used to trim the beak of the birds in order to prevent pecking and also to reduce feed loss. It is generally used in layer farm. It is of two types - manual and electrical beak trimmer. Electrical debeaker is usually mounted on to a stand of convenient height (0.60 to 0.75 m) with a peddle connected to the top of the unit with a chain. When the operator presses the peddle with his/her foot, the hot blade slides down cutting the beak placed over a small platform in the equipment.

viii) **Heating equipment :** In regions where extreme cold weather conditions are experienced, electric room heaters are employed to maintain comfortable room temperature for the birds. However, in north India, Bukhari is commonly used in winters inside the poultry sheds to keep birds warm during nights. Bukhari is a traditional heat generating equipment made up of a burning chamber for burning wood or saw dust with a chimney at the top. However, the major disadvantage is that it generates poisonous gases and may results in huge deaths of birds if used in a closed room.

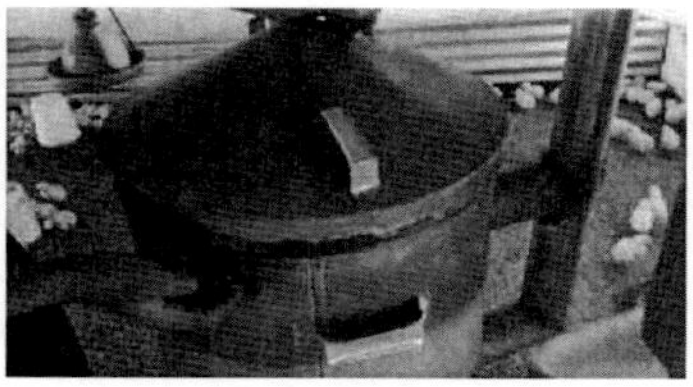

Bukhari

ix) **Refrigerator :** A refrigerator is essential in a poultry farm for storing vaccines and other medicines.

x) **Shovel and raking tool :** Shovel is used in poultry farms for removal of manure. Raking tool is made up of iron rod with sharp projections fitted with iron or wooden handle. In broiler farms, where the birds are maintained on deep litter system, raking tool is used for raking or mixing the litter to prevent cake formation and to keep the litter dry. If raking is not done regularly, bird's droppings will mix with the litter material resulting in cake formation.

xi) **Sprayers :** Sprayers are used for disinfection of building, birds, men, material and surrounding areas. Though different types of sprayers are available in the market, hand-operated sprayers which can be carried on the back are the most ideal for poultry farm operations.

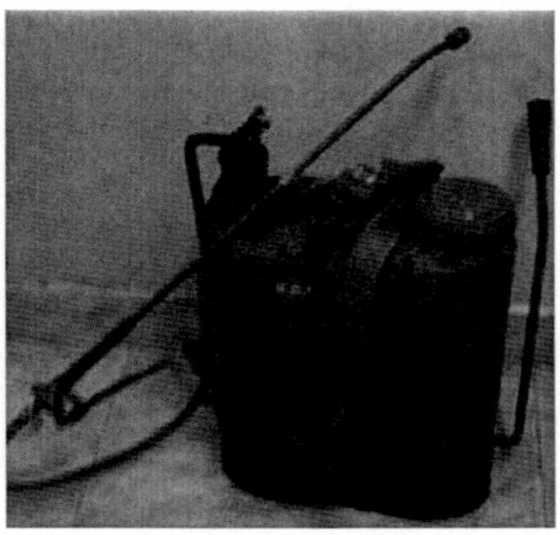

Sprayer

xii) **Sprinklers and foggers :** Sprinklers and foggers are used to provide cooling effect to the birds in hot dry weather conditions. Whereas, in hot-humid conditions, commercial irrigation sprinklers should be used only on the roof tops during afternoon hours. If very hot weather is expected, foggers can be used to spray fine mist of water directly only on the face of the birds. Since the feathers are water-proof, foggers should not be used to wet the feathers.

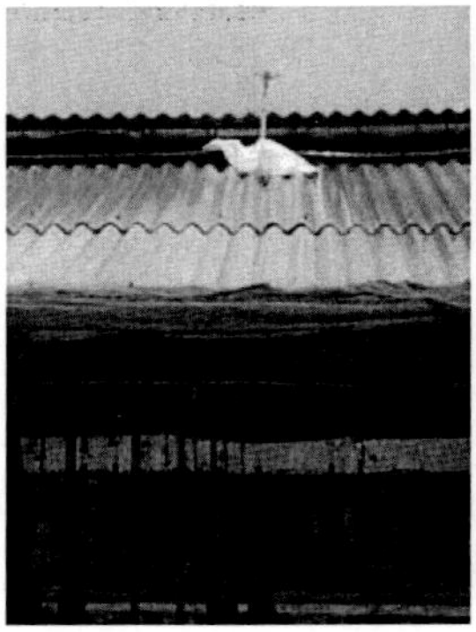

Sprinkler on the roof top

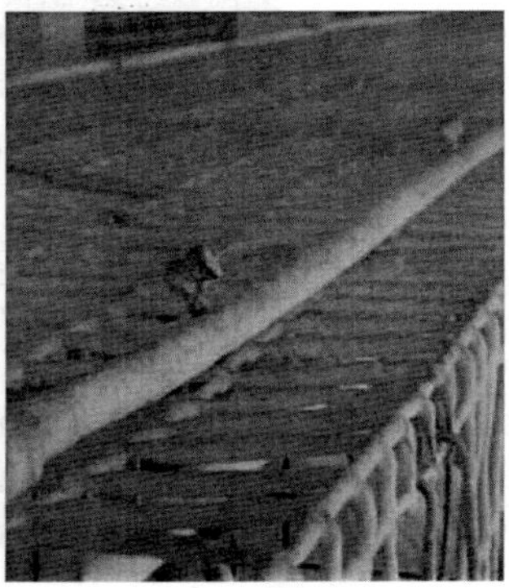

Fogger over the cage

xiii) **Thermometer :** It is a small device used for measuring temperature. Most commonly used thermometer in the poultry shed are wet and dry bulb thermometers used for measuring temperature and humidity.

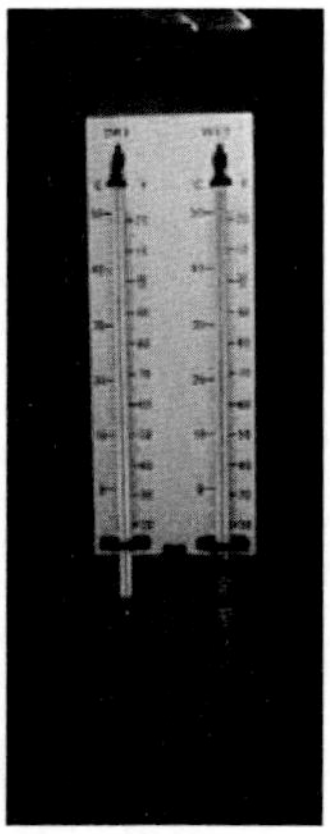

Wet and Dry bulb Thermometers

xiv) **Trolley :** A small vehicle with two or four wheels operated manually to transport cages/crates and other heavy objects from one place to another.

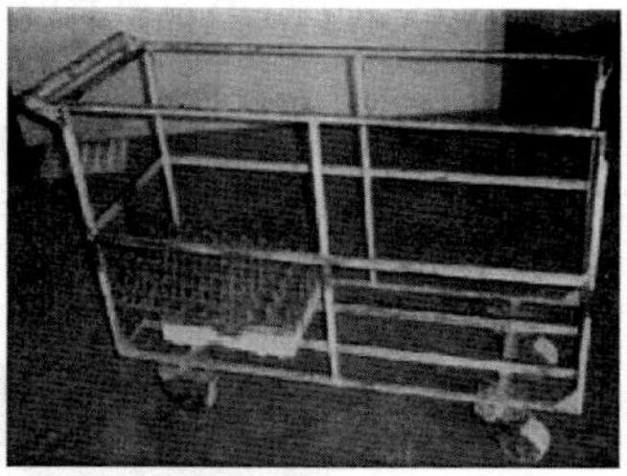

Trolley

xv) **Weighing balance :** Weighing balance is used for weighing of the birds and feed. Now-a-days, balance with a digital display is available at affordable price. If a farmer wishes to sell broilers on retail, a 5 kg or 1 kg balance is required. However, if the birds are sold wholesale, a spring balance or plateform balance with a sensitivity of 100 or 25 g is advisable.

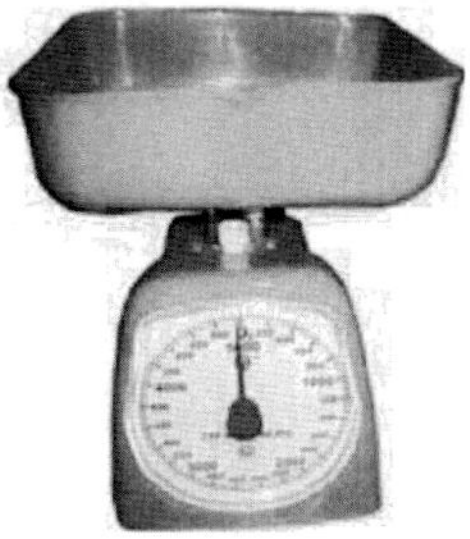

Weighing Balance

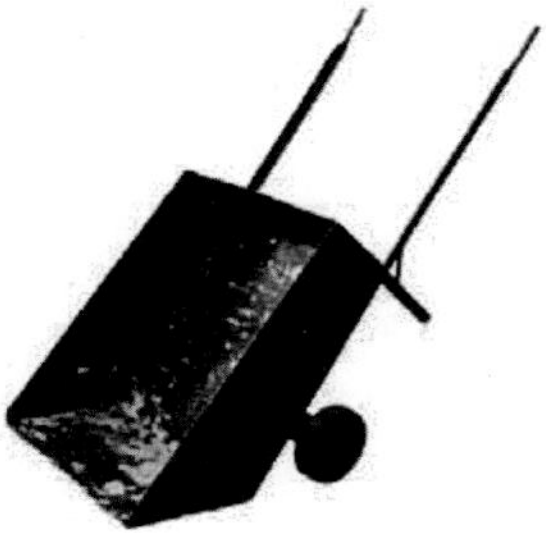

Wheel Barrow

xvi) **Wheel barrow :** It is small hand operated vehicle with a single wheel in the front and two supporting legs and two handles at the back. It is used to carrying poultry farm waste from the shed to the place of disposal.

□□□

Chapter 8

Management of Chicks and Broilers

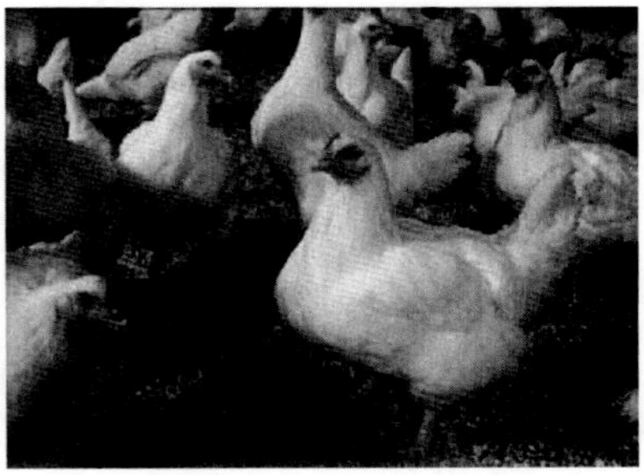

Broiler production is quite different from layer production. With margins so small, the producer, whether a small farmer or an integrator must be aware of the many factors that affect the cost of production. Although each factor exerts only a minor influence, the combined effect of all factors becomes phenomenal in the broiler management.

General characteristics

A broiler is a young chicken of either sex, raised purely for meat purposes. They achieve marketable weight of 1.8-2.0 Kg usually by 6-7 weeks of age. This is on account of their fast growth; high feed conversion efficiency, good conformation and early feathering.

In Broiler production, the birds, their nutritional requirements, housing and environmental requirements, management, processing and marketing of final produce are all different than their counterpart used for egg production. However, basic principles of poultry production in brooding may be similar. Hence, the basic knowledge of poultry production can be utilized with modifications for efficient production of meat.

The broiler chicks should be purchased from a reputed hatchery that provides pullorum-typhoid free clean chicks. The qualities of a good broiler chick are:

1. Fast growth
2. Good livability

3. Fast feathering
4. Uniformity
5. Good feed conversion efficiency.

Achievement of the genetic potential inherent in the birds depends upon making sure that all the factors related the broiler production are given full and correct attention. All of these are interdependent. If any one of these elements is suboptimal, then overall broiler performance will suffer.

Rearing Systems

Broilers are generally reared by following two systems:

I. All-in, all-out system

This system means that all chicks of similar age are placed in the house at the same time, reared and then disposed off also at the same time. This programme is, therefore, called "all-in, all-out" and is much more successful. All the premises are then thoroughly cleaned, disinfected and rested. This provides a period when there are no chicks in the shed. This breaks any disease cycle at the farm.

II. Multiple Age group system

In this system, chicks of different age groups are reared at the same farm. This system of rearing is difficult to manage and disease outbreaks.

Management of Chicks

The management of chicks includes the brooding and rearing which is the care and management of young chicks after hatching. The care and management of chicks during initial part of their life constitutes brooding. Successful brooding will lead to the production of healthy birds for meat production called as Broilers.

The following mangemental steps should be considered during rearing of broiler chicks:

a) Preparations before the arrival of chicks
b) Management after the arrival of chicks

a) Before the arrival of chicks

Before the arrival of chicks, you need to make suitable arrangements, which are as follows:

1. Brooder house should be cleaned and disinfected.
2. Feeders and drinkers should be cleaned and disinfected followed by sundrying.
3. House must be thoroughly examined for leaking roof and gutters, drafty doors, functioning of fans, switchboards, shutters, etc. The floor may be given a coat of lime solution.
4. Floor of the building has to be cleaned with a suitable detergent and disinfected with a commercial product suitable for floor cleaning.
5. All weeds and debris, if any, surrounding the building must be cleared and the area sprayed with a commercial disinfectant.
6. Check the brooders, feeders, drinkers and other equipment which are required during the brooding period.
7. New and clean, dry, mould-free absorbent litter should be spread evenly on the floor to a thickness of about 6 to 8 cm; care has to be taken not to close all the windows, when the litter is being spread so that dust can settle down easily.
8. Paper is spread on the litter.
9. Brooder, feeders and drinkers should be arranged at least 6 to 8 hours before the arrival of chicks; brooder should be put on so that requisite brooder temperature is attained before the arrival of chicks; if required, windows may have to be covered with gunny bags to conserve heat. This also helps to maintain drinking water temperature at 18°C.
10. The feeders should be arranged in the brooding area like spokes in a wheel; with half the length of the feeders inside the canopy area. The drinkers should be arranged at the edge of the canopy interspersed between the feeders. This is done to ensure both feed and water within 30 cm (1 ft) of distance from any part of the brooding area, especially at the beginning of brooding. Later on, both feeders and drinkers should be uniformly distributed so that no bird need move more than 3 m to have access of either feed or water.

11. Anti-stress factors (B-complex vitamins, vitamin C, etc.) may be added in water.
12. Feed or maize grit should be sprinkled on paper to help chicks identify the feed. During the first few days, it is mandatory that the chicks should have feed available easily. Therefore, the feed should be kept in inverted chick box lids, egg flats or any such large flat containers.

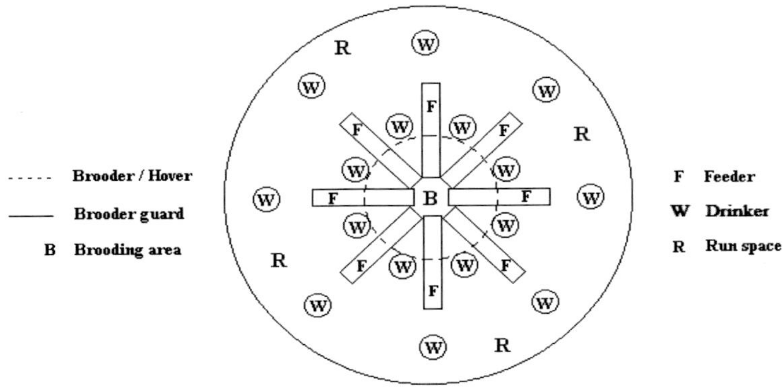

Arrangement of equipment during brooding

13. It is desirable to have a standby sawdust bukhari otherwise, a charcoal bukhari, kerosene or LPG must be available to meet emergencies in case of power failure.
14. All data sheets required for recording various events like medication, vaccination, feed consumption, mortality, etc. should be kept ready.

b) After the arrival of chicks

Release of chicks

1. It is advisable to examine a sample of chicks from each of the chick boxes to ascertain the quality and thriftiness of the chicks; it also helps to note mortality, if any, during transit.
2. It is a good practice to dip the beaks of the newly hatched chicks in water at drinkers and leave them into the brooder area. Otherwise, the chick box can be inverted quickly to dump all the chicks nearby the brooding area.
3. Chicks should be observed carefully to identify weak ones and also to help those which are not able to reach feed and water.

4. It is equally necessary to observe and ensure that all the chicks are actually eating and watch out for "starve-outs" by examining randomly for well-distended crop (a pouch just below the base of the neck, which can be felt by gentle pressing on the area).

Brooding

Providing additional heat to chicks after hatching is called Brooding. Brooding period is generally for 4 weeks and can be extended, if the outside temperature is too low and vice versa.

Systems of Brooding

Systems of brooding refer to the methods of applying heat to the chicks during brooding period.

The following are the main four methods of brooding:

1. **Hot room brooding :** in this method, the entire brooder room is heated through central heating system. The central heating is achieved by one of the several methods like circulating hot water in pipes or under floor heating or blowing air -type. The system makes the ventilation easier in brooder house and keeps the litter free from dampness.
2. **Cold room brooding :** It involves heating only a limited area using a canopy. A canopy is hung down from the roof with the edge of the canopy about 8 to 10 cm above the litter floor. This facilitates movement of chicks in and out of the brooder at will. Bulbs are fixed inside the canopy. These bulbs heat the surrounding air and by convection, the air within the brooder is heated.

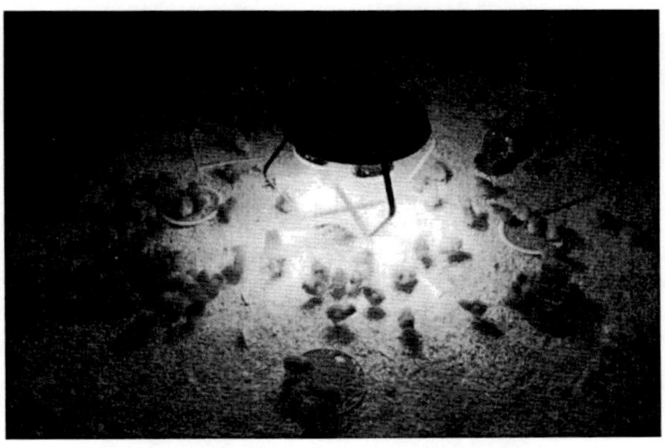

Cold room brooding of chicks

Wattage and number of bulbs fixed inside a canopy depends on the outside temperature and number of birds under the canopy. Generally, two or three 40 or 60 W incandescent bulbs are used inside a canopy. The canopy is raised as the birds grow and removed after the requisite brooding period.

Number of canopy brooders

- Broiler chicks require 75 and 150 sq cm of brooding and run space, respectively.
- For 1000 chicks, it is advisable to have four canopy brooders of 120 cm diameter at one brooder for every 250 chicks.
- For broiler chicks, one brooder is required for every 200 chicks.

3. Battery brooder : The brooding can be done in batteries also. Brooding in batteries is popular in commercial farms. Usually mortality is less in batteries than in floor brooding. The birds remain free of coccidiosis. Labour requirement is less in this system.

Brooding requirements

Temperature

Chicks hatched out require supplementary heat till they grow feathers. It is not possible to specify the exact brooding temperature for all the conditions; it depends largely upon environmental temperature and general conditions of chicks. Under low environmental temperature, chicks appear to be comfortable at higher temperature vice –versa, Similarly chicks under stress of any kind also need higher brooder temperature. If the brooding temperature is correct, the chicks will move uniformly in both brooder area as well as run space. At the beginning, a temperature of 35°C (95°F) is provided which is reduced at a rate of 2.8°C (5°F) per week till the end of brooding. If temperature is not reduced, stepwise, thermoregulatory mechanism will not develop properly and feather growth will be severely affected. Therefore, brooding temperature is reduced at a rate of 2.8°C (5°F) per week till the end of brooding period.

Table 1: The temperature requirement for chicks during different weeks

Age in weeks	Temperature under hover at 5 cm above floor in °C/°F
0-1	35 / 95
1-2	32 / 90
2-3	29 / 85
3-4	26 / 80
4-5	23 / 75

Measuring the brooding temperature

Brooding temperature of 35°C is warm for humans and we start sweating slightly inside a brooder house; i.e. in the beginning of brooding, if we feel uncomfortable, the birds will be comfortable (this is referred to as "Chicken sense" of the farmer). However, if measured by a thermometer, it is placed at a height of 8 to 10 cm above the litter floor under the brooder (in case of reflector brooder and infra-red bulbs) and at the edge of the canopy in case of canopy brooding. As the birds grow in size, the height at which temperature is measured should also be increased. Measurement should be made at a height where most part of the body is held while standing (i.e. other than head, neck and legs) is likely to be present.

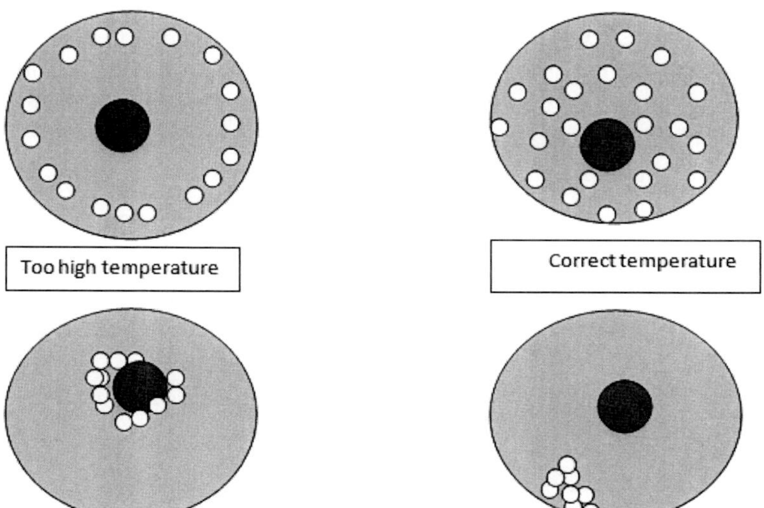

Indication of correct brooding temperature

This is particularly important during the first 8 to 10 days of age because:

1. The paper prevents eating of the litter material by the chicks because they can't identify the feed yet. If they eat paddy husk, they are likely to die due to choking. Feed sprinkled on the paper will be easily visible for the chicks to identify and eat.
2. Paper on the litter also helps observe the birds undisturbed, paper is spread on the litter and is turned after 4 to 5 days and removed after 8 to 10 days. Question comes how the paper helps observation of chicks.

Distribution of fecal matter in and around the brooder is the indicator of brooding comfort and if paper is not spread, the fecal matter mixes with the litter material. It is interesting that when cold wind blows from right hand side, probably due to leakage through curtains (drafty), the birds lean on the brooder guards.

a) Ventilation: Fresh air is important for good health and well being of chicks. Three to five air changes per hour are ample. Poor ventilation results in accumulation of carbon dioxide, carbon monoxide and ammonia which leads to wet litter. Concentration of carbon monoxide more than 0.01 per cent becomes poisonous to chicks. Obnoxious odour of ammonia irritates the eyes of chicks and retards the body growth. Wet litter due to poor ventilation is often predisposing factor for outbreak of coccidiosis, the extent of ventilation is governed by the condition of litter. There should be enough ventilation to keep the litter dry.

b) Humidity : Though the range of humidity requirement for floor brooded chicks have been shown to be wide (30% TO 75%) too low or too high humidity in brooder house should be avoided. High humidity creates the problem of wet litter, which the development of coccidiosis. Low humidity may cause dusty litter resulting in respiratory trouble and poor growth of feathers. Fifty to sixty per cent of relative humidity is proper in floor type brooder house.

c) Floor space : Brooder space of 45-65 square cm per chick is recommended. A hover of 1.8 metres diameter can accommodate 500 chicks. However, the number of chicks brooded under the hover should be as per the manufactures. When small pens are used for brooding, dimension of the house should be taken into consideration for brooding the number of chicks. On floor brooding provide 1 square ft. floor area per chick till 6 weeks of age.

A. Feeding Management

Broiler chicken requires different level of nutrients. In this regard, broiler chickens are fed the following three types of diets:

- Broiler Pre-starter ration is fed from 0-10days of age.
- Broiler Starter ration is fed from 11-25days of age.
- Broiler Finisher ration is fed from 26-35 days of age.

Table 2: Nutrient Requirements of Broiler chicken

Type of feed	Age (Days)	Crude Protein (%)	Metabolizable Energy (Kcal/kg)	Crude Fibre Max (%)	Calcium (%)	Phosphorus (%)
Pre-Starter	0-10	23	2900	6	1	0.5
Starter	11-25	22	3000	6	1	0.5
Finisher	26-42	21	3100	6	1	0.5

Broiler chicken should be provided these diets ad lib. The feed consumption during different weeks in birds is given below:

Table 3: Feed consumption of Broilers

Age (weeks)	Feed consumption		
	g/bird/d	kg/bird/week	Cumulative (kg)
1	16.8	0.12	0.12
2	41.4	0.41	0.41
3	65.0	0.86	0.86
4	90.5	1.49	1.49
5	115.0	2.30	2.30
6	143.7	3.29	3.29
7	170.9	4.49	4.49
8	188.2	5.80	5.80

The broiler rations are prepared by mixing different feed ingredients in a required ratio so as to formulate a complete balanced ration to be fed to birds during different stages of life.

Table 4: Suggested Rations for Broilers

Ingredients (kg/100kg)	Starter		Finisher	
	1	2	1	2
Maize	43.75	57.10	65.10	44.10
Rice polish	10.00	-	-	20.00
Groundnut-cake	14.00	-	-	11.00
Sunflower cake	14.00	15.00	12.00	11.00
Mustard-cake (solvent-extracted)	-	10.00	10.00	-
Fish meal (43% protein)	10.00	6.00	5.00	5.50
Meat meal (56% protein)	-	7.00	5.00	5.50
Silkworm pupae-meal (40% protein)	3.50	3.00	1.20	-
Animal fat	3.00	1.00	-	1.25
Bone-meal	1.15	-	0.60	0.60
Limestone	-	0.50	0.60	0.70
Salt	0.50	0.30	0.40	0.25
Mineral * and vitamin ** mixture	0.10	0.10	0.10	0.10
Total	100.00	100.00	100.00	100.00

A standard chart can be adopted for observing the weekly growth performance of broilers.

Table 5: Standard chart for observing weekly growth performance of Broilers

Age in weeks	Avg B.wt(g)	Feed intake/1000birds(g)	Feed efficiency	Water intake 1000 birds/day(lit)
0	42	----	----	----
1	170	19	0.86	46
2	380	37	1.12	89
3	720	68	1.31	165

4	1170	102	1.48	245
5	1680	134	1.62	320
6	2220	168	1.80	405

Water management

1. Provide at least 30 drinkers per 1000 birds.
2. Minimum water space per bird should be:

   1 inch upto 4 weeks

   2 inches after 4 weeks

   One round drinker for 50 birds
3. Usually a bird drinks 2-3 litres of water for each Kg of feed it consumes. However, this depends on the weather conditions. It is, therefore, very important that fresh clean water always available by providing adequate number of drinkers. Water intake increases by 2-3 times during summer months.

Light Management

Lighting and how it is managed (hours of light and dark and how light is distributed throughout the day) can impact on both broiler productivity and welfare. Broilers benefit from having a definite pattern of light and dark (day and night) creating distinct periods of rest and activity. A number of important physiological and behavioural processes follow normal diurnal rhythms. Therefore, defined cycles of light and dark allow broilers to experience natural patterns of growth, development and behaviour.

Light adjustment is used in the broiler house to increase growth, improve feed efficiency, decrease mortality and reduce electricity costs.

1. It is advisable to provide continuous (23 hours light: 1 hours dark per day) during the entire cycle.
2. After two weeks, the lights can be dimmed to reduce the activity of the birds. Thus, the weight gain is higher.

There are four important components to lighting programme. These are:

- Photoperiod length - The number of hours of light and dark given in a 24 hours period.
- Photoperiod distribution— How the hours of light and dark are distributed throughout 24 hour period.
- Wave length—Colour of light
- Light intensity—How bright the light provided is.

Light Duration and Pattern

The lighting programme used by many broiler growers in the past has been to provide what is essentially continuous lighting (a long continuous light period, followed by a short dark of up to an hour). The belief was that if lights were continuously on, birds would eat and drink more, and grow faster. This assumption is not correct. Continuous light causes depressed body weights and has negative impact on broiler health and welfare as well. After 7 days of age around 5 hours of darknesss may be optimum (4-6 hours). There is no reduction in growth rate to 39 days and possibly an increase to 49 days of age. Feed conversion efficiency improves particularly in the latter stages of growth. Bird morbidity is improved and the severity of footpad lesions may be reduced. The proportion of meat as leg meat may be increased.

The degree to which a lighting programme will effect broiler production is influenced by a number of factors as:

- The time of program implementation: Early implementation being most effective benefits health of birds.
- Age at processing: Older birds being likely to benefit more from darkness exposure.
- Environment: The effects of increased stocking density will be made worse by longer darkness exposure.
- Feeder management: The effects of limited feeder space will be made worst by longer darkness exposure.
- Rate of bird growth: The impact of lighting will be greater in rapidly growing birds.

All lighting programs should provide for long daylenght, such as 23 hours light and I hour dark in the early stages of growth—up to 7 days of age. It is recommended that a minimum 4 hours of darkness should be provided from 7 days of age.

Light colour and Source

Several types of light sources can be used for broilers. The most common types of lighting are incandescent, florescent or LED.

- Incandescent lights provide a good special range but are not energy efficient.
- Fluorescent lights are more efficient than incandescent lights but lose intensity over time and must be replaced before actually failing.
- LED (Light emitting diodes) lighting is efficient and specific lighting colours can be chosen. Initial cost is high but bulbs last much longer.

Light Intensity

A light intensity of 30-40 lux (3-4 fc) from 0-7 days of age and at least 5-10 lux (0.5-1.0 fc) therefore, will improve feeding activity and growth. A low daytime light intensity (below 5 lux/0.5fc) may have negative impacts on mortality. FCR and growth. Low light intensities may also:

- Affect eye growth
- Lead to increased footpad lesions
- Reduce activity and comfort behaviour.
- Impact on physiological rthymus as birds may not be able to detect the difference between day and night.

Litter Management

The most commonly used litters are sawdust, rice husk and wood shavings. Litter should be fresh, dry and free from moulds.

Different types of litter materials are available depending on the geographical region having different advantages and disadvantages.

Table 6: Different types of Litter materials

Litter Materials	Advantages / Disadvantages
Saw dust and Pine shavings	Preferred litter material in many areas Becoming expensive and limited in supply
Hardwood shavings and Saw-dust	Often high in moisture Can become susceptible to dangerous mold growth
Pine or Hardwood chips	Used successfully in many areas May cause an increase in breast blisters, if allowed to become too wet.
Pine or Hardwood bark	Similar to chips and shavings in moisture holding capacity Medium sized particles are preferred.
Rice Hulls	A good litter material where available at a competitive price. Young chicks may be prone to litter eating.
Peanut Hulls	An inexpensive litter material in peat nut producing areas Does have tendency to cake and crust. Some problems with pesticides has been noticed
Coconut Husks	An inexpensive litter material in coconut producing areas. Does not have the tendency to cake.
Sand	Can be used in arid areas on concrete floors. If too deep bird movement may be impeded. Needs good management. More difficult to maintain floor temperature during cold weather brooding. Need ample time and ventilation prior to brooding to ensure dryness.
Crushed corn cobs	Limited availability May cause increased incidence of breast blisters
Chopped Straw or Hay	High incidence of caking Mold growth is possible Best used 50/50 with wood shaving
Straw Pellets	Increased water holding capacity Cakes less easily than sawdust
Processed Paper	Can be difficult to manage in humid areas Tendency to cake with increased particle size Top dressing paper base with shavings may be helpful to decrease caking
Chemically Treated Straw Pellets	Must be used as recommended by the supplier
Peat Mass	Can be successfully used
Flax Straw	Low incidence of caking Not dusty Good absorption
Recycled Litter	Not recommended Increased incidence of bacterial contamination

No matter what type of litter material is used in the broiler farm, good litter should provide:

- Good moisture absorption
- Biodegradability
- Bird comfort
- Low dust level
- Freedom from contamination
- Consistent availability from a biosecure source
- Concrete floors are washable and allow for more effective biosecurity and litter management.

Poor litter quality is an influential factor in the increased incidence of footpad dermatitis (FFD). Since the primary cause of FFD is wet and caked litter, it is important to maintain the proper ventilation for moisture control in the house. FFD may cause an increased incidence of carcass downgrading and should be monitored to determine, if additional litter needs to be added.

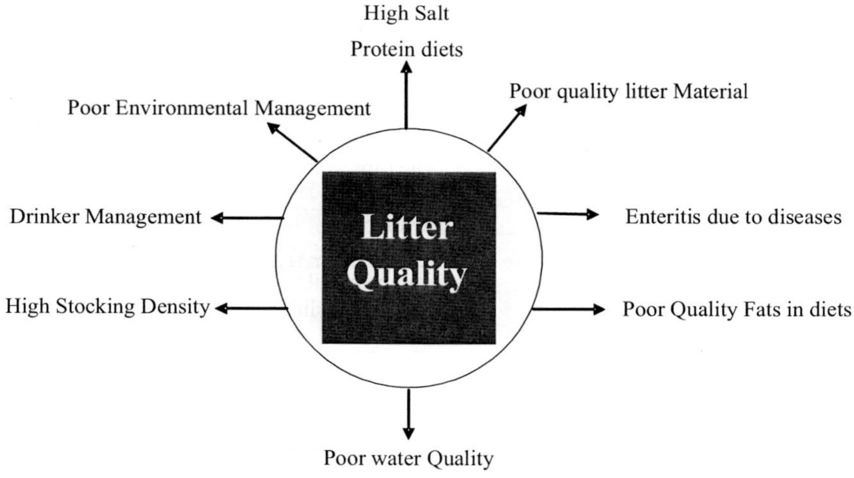
High Salt
Protein diets
Poor quality litter Material
Poor Environmental Management
Drinker Management
Litter Quality
Enteritis due to diseases
High Stocking Density
Poor Quality Fats in diets
Poor water Quality

Causes of poor quality litter

- In the well managed farms, the litter is neither too dusty nor too wet. The litter that has correct moisture (20-25%) adheres slightly and breaks up, when dropped from the hand. When litter contains an excess of moisture, it balls up (i.e., forms into a ball) in the hands, when squeezed and when dry it does not adhere.

- Avoid spillage of water. It will cause wet litter problem. At least twice weekly, rake the litter up gently and remove moist lumps, cakes, etc.
- Apply hydrated lime powder at the rate of 0.5Kg per 10 Sq. ft. area during the raking to keep the litter dry and odour free. Do not use unhydrated lime powder, as it is an irritant. Also, do not rake the dry litter, as this will lead to dust problem that may predispose to respiratory diseases.

Role of a Manger in the Broiler Production

The objective of the broiler manager is to achieve the required flock performance in terms of bird welfare, live weight, feed conversion efficiency, uniformity and meat yield within economic constraints. Broiler production is a sequential process with ultimate performance being dependent on each step being completed successfully. For maximum performance to be attained, each stage must be assessed critically and improvement made wherever required.

The complexity of broiler production means that livestock managers should have a clear understanding of the factors affecting whole production process as well as of those directly influencing bird management on the farm. Changes may also be necessary in the hatchery, during transport and in the processing plant. Within broiler production, there are several stages of development of the bird as the bird moves from egg, to farm and then the processing plant. Between each of these stages in the production process is a transition phase. Transition must be managed with minimum bird stress. The key transitions from the broiler producer are:

- Chick hatching
- Take off, storage and transportation of chick
- Development of a good feeding behaviour in young chicks
- Change over from supplementary feeding and drinking system
- Catching and transport of the broiler at depletion.

The importance of a farm manager must not be under estimated. A good farm manager should be able to identify and respond to problems quickly. A farm manager must be constantly in tune with and aware of the birds in the flock and their environment. To do this, the bird's behaviour characteristics and the conditions within the poultry house must be closely observed. This monitoring is commonly referred to as stock sense and is continuous process that uses aii the stockman's senses.

Slowly enter the house and stop until the birds become accustomed to your presence. During this time, continuously use all your senses to assess the flock condition. LOOK, LISTEN, SMELL AND FEEL.

Look at

- Bird distribution over the floor area: Are specific areas being avoided?
- Bird respiration : Are the birds panting? Is the panting specific to one area of the shed suggesting an airflow or temperature issue?
- Bird behaviour-feeding, drinking and resting: Normally broilers will be evenly split between these behaviours.
- Litter condition : Are areas capping due to leaking drinkers or excess water from cool areas? Is cold air entering the shed and falling to the floor?
- Feeders and drinkers : Are they of right height? Is there feed in the feeders? Are the drinkers leaking? What is feed quality like?

Listen to

- The birds : Are the birds sneezing or making respiratory noise changes? What are their vocalizations like? Is it related to a dusty or poor environment?
- The feeders : Are the mechanical augers constantly running?
- The fans : Are the fan bearing noisy? Do the fan belts sound loose? Routine maintenance can prevent environmental issues related to suboptimal air quality.

Feel

- The air : How does the air feel on your face? Stuffy, cold, hot, fast air speed, no air speed?

- The feed physical quality : Is the crumb very dusty? Do the pellets break down very easily in the hands and in the feeder?
- The litter condition : Pick up and feel the condition. If the litter stays together after compressing, which indicates excessive moisture which suggests poor ventilation.

Smell

- The feed : What does the feed smell like? Does it smell fresh or musty?
- The environment : What does the environment smell like? Can you smell ammonia?

Individual birds may be assessed for the following symptoms:

- Eyes should be clear, no signs of irritation.
- Skin should be unblemished with no scratches or hock burn marks.
- Breast should be unblemished with no blisters.
- Feathering should be clean with no feathers sticking out.
- Leg health. What is the gait of the birds?
- Feet and hocks should be clean with no irritation markings.
- Vent should be clean with no signs of loose dropping.
- Beak and tongue should have no nasal discharge and no signs of tongue discolouration.
- Crop. Are they feeding? Does the crop contain litter? Is the crop very hard or soft? This will indicate the availability of water.
- General demeanor and alertness.

❑❑❑

Chapter **9**

Management of Growers

There are Three Stages in Layer Farming:

1. Chick stage (chicks) 1-8 weeks
2. Growing stage (growers) 9-18 weeks
3. Layer stage (layers) 9 weeks onward, usually up to 72 weeks

1. Chick stage

This stage can also be called as "brooding stage" and birds during this period are called "chicks". The management in this stage is already discussed earlier in "Management of broiler chicken" chapter.

2. Growing stage

The period, after brooding up to sexual maturity, is called "growing period" and birds during this stage are referred to as "growers".

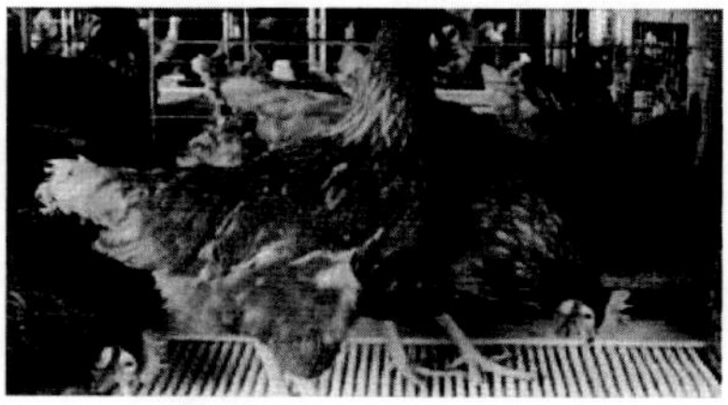

Grower birds on slat system

Both chick and the growing stage are great importance for the future performance of the layer bird. It is during these two phases that the correct body weight and uniformity are obtained, which shape the future performance of the adult bird.

The growing period follows the brooding period. Probably no other age of chicken commands the respect of the management more than the period between the time they are 6-8 weeks of age and sexual maturity. How well a bird is grown will greatly determine how well it does in laying or breeding house..The chicks now are 8 weeks old and they are sufficiently hardy. They are not yet ready to produce eggs; they need a different managerial approach to make them perform to their best during the next period, the laying period. The growing female birds are also referred to as "Pullets"; pullet is a female chicken under 1 year of age and has not yet started laying eggs.

During growing period, the routine works of feeding, offering of water, litter management, healthcare and maintenance of records are continued. However, suitable changes are made considering the floor, feeder and drinker space requirement. In addition to these, the birds will be subjected to feed restriction and trimming of beaks during this period.

Routine Management

Floor space

Floor space required upto 16 weeks is 900 sq cm (1 sq ft) per bird and the Brood – Grow House (BGH) has the required space. However, for brooding, only a part of bird is increased the space should have been. Hence, the birds are distributed to the entire area so that the birds receive optimum space to move around freely.

Feeder space

Feeder space required per to 6 cm from 4 cm. Circular feeders for growers will be slightly bigger and will have a diameter of 42 cm. That means, a feeder space of 132 cm is available, which is adequate for about 28 to 29 growers (say 30 birds). For 1000 growers, about 35 feeders are required. Linear feeders are not commonly used for growers.

Feeders are arranged at the level of the back of birds as done for chicks till 8 weeks. They are filled as and when feed gets exhausted; generally every 4 to 5 days.

Drinker space

Drinker space required is 2 cm per bird (1.5 cm per bird up to 8 weeks of age). Bell type drinkers of 35 cm diameter are used. Each of such drinkers provides 110 cm of drinker space and is adequate for 71 to 72 birds (say 70 birds). For 1000 birds, about 15 such bell type drinkers are required.

Bell type drinkers also are arranged at the level of the back of birds.

Litter management

Same as outlined under "Management of Chicks".

Lighting management

Specific lighting programs is recommended during growing period. But, in the houses where sidewalls are made of expanded metal, light control is not possible. Therefore, the general practice is not to provide any artificial light during this period.

Feed Restriction

Quantity of feed to be offered at different ages to growers is given by the supplier of the laying type of chicks. It is less than the quantity of feed the birds would consume, if they are allowed to consume as much as they want (*ad libitum*). That means, amount of feed given is restricted; i.e. Feed Restriction.

Advantages

1. If the growing birds are fed *ad libitum*, they tend to become heavy and obese (fatty).
2. Excessive body weight is also associated with reduced disease resistance and hence, feed restricted birds are likely to survive better.
3. More ova will be released at a time (multiple ovulations), which results in smaller eggs at the beginning of egg production which can't be sold. Hence, number of saleable eggs is reduced.
4. A considerable saving on feed cost can be achieved because, only about 92 to 93% of the calculated feed requirement will be offered.
5. They are likely to consume less feed per dozen eggs even during laying period, when they are offered *ad libitum* feed.
6. The pullets accumulate less fat and therefore, produce more eggs.
7. It is easier to identify weaker birds at an early age during feed restriction. Culling of such birds helps not only saving feed but also promoting layer house survivability because, healthier birds will be moving to layer house.
8. Layers feed restricted during growing period have been found to produce heavier eggs in longer clutches than those fed *ad libitum*.

Disadvantages

1. Feed restricted birds mature late; but this is more than compensated by sustained production of heavier eggs. Overall, more and heavier eggs are produced.
2. Because of restricted feed, there will be competition for eating feed. Consequent on this, weaker birds become weak further and can be easily identified and removed by the farmer or they may even die. Therefore, grower house survivability reduces.

30 Feed-restriction requires technical supervision.

Methods

Feed restriction can be effected by several ways like:

1. Quantitative feed restriction – offering 92-93% (commercial egg-type pullets) of the calculated feed requirement / skip-a-day program in which the birds are fed on alternate days from 9 weeks to sexual maturity. Once a pullet lays her first egg; she is referred to as a "Layer".
2. Increasing fibre content which increases bulk in the intestine thereby reducing feed intake. If fibre content is increased, by using ingredients like wheat bran, rice bran, etc., the birds eat less.
3. Reducing protein content. Proteins are highly essential for growth. Therefore, reduced protein content delays growth and, in turn, sexual maturity.
4. Reducing lysine content. Lysine is very essential for growth. Thus, reduction in lysine is same as reducing protein content.
5. Reduction in energy content (similar to increasing fibre).

Under commercial conditions, quantitative feed restriction is commonly practiced on egg-type pullets mainly because it is easier to practice and the chick-supplier will be providing a readymade chart of the quantity of feed to be offered during the growing period.

Effects of feed restriction

1. Delays onset of sexual maturity (age at which 50% of the birds are producing eggs or average of the age at which each of the birds produces her first egg) from a few days to 3-4 weeks depending on severity of restriction.

2. Reduces the body weight of the bird at sexual maturity, usually by reduction in body fat.
3. May lead to certain nutritional deficiency / ies.
4. Although cost of raising a pullet is reduced, the additional time required to reach sexual maturity would nullify such benefits.
5. Generally, livability (or survivability) during egg production improves.
6. Egg production is not generally affected.
7. Egg weight normally improves because of delayed sexual maturity. Egg weight is dependant directly on yolk (yellow part of the egg) weight. Yolk comes directly from ovaries by accumulation over a period of time. Therefore, as age at sexual maturity increases, more yolk material is accumulated thereby weight of yolk increases.
8. In the layer house, birds tend to consume less feed per dozen eggs. This is a matter of habit; the layers are forced to consume less than their maximum during growing period. Therefore, they tend to consume less during laying period as well.

Body weight during feed restriction

It is recommended that the body weights of the pullets be maintained as shown below on the weekly schedule beginning from 7/8 weeks of age. It must be remembered that egg-type pullets, being smaller, are more sensitive to feed restriction; therefore, they do not respond positively for any feed restriction in excess of 7-8%. A sample of birds must be weighed regularly during the growing period to ensure desired growth rate.

Table 1: Feed intake by Grower birds

Age (wks)	Average Body weight (g)	Average Feed consumption g/bird/week	Cumulative feed consumption g/bird
1	65	92.4	
2	121	114.1	206.5
3	186	171.5	378.0
4	262	222.6	600.6
5	335	254.1	854.7
6	427	266.7	1121.4
7	513	273.0	1394.4

8	593	286.3	1680.7
9	671	301.7	1982.4
10	754	317.8	2300.2
11	828	333.9	2634.1
12	904	349.3	2983.4
13	968	365.4	3348.8
14	1030	381.5	3730.3
15	1092	397.6	4127.9
16	1157	413.0	4540.9
By the end of 16 weeks	1157	4540.9	
Note: Assuming that average chick weight at hatch is 37 g, weight gain till 16 weeks is (1157 – 37) = 1120 g for which each bird has consumed 4540.9 g of feed. Therefore, feed consumed per kg weigh gain (referred to as Feed Conversion Ratio, FCR) = (4540.9 ÷ 1120) = 4.054 or approximately 4.0.			

Beak Trimming (Debeaking)

This is popularly known as debeaking. The term "Debeaking" literally means removal of beaks; but it involves the partial removal of the upper and lower beak. Therefore, "Beak trimming" is a better nomenclature. It is undertaken usually after 6 weeks of age and most often in the grower house. It can be done in the brooder house also. It is performed by using an electrically heated blade. (De-beaker)

Why beak trimming is performed?

The reasons why beak trimming is performed is as follows:

1. A group of birds (flock) in an enclosure (called "Pen") will develop its own social order (peck order) depending on dominance amongst the birds. For this, they may resort to fighting as well. This may lead to injury, bleeding and cannibalism.
2. Some birds develop some vices (bad habits) like feather pulling, vent (anus) pecking, etc. This might again result in bleeding and cannibalism.
3. Avoid feed wastage.
   a) Quantitative: Birds have a natural tendency to scratch the feed and search for grains especially when feed is in the mash form. In the process, there will be spillage of feed out of the feeders.

   b) Qualitative: Birds do establish a peck order within the pen. The stronger birds access feed first and preferentially pick and eat the grains (also a natural instinct), if beaks are not trimmed.

All animals primarily eat to satisfy energy needs. It is well known that the grains are energy-rich but poor in all other nutrients. Therefore, stronger birds will get satisfied with less quantity of grains. Hence, the stronger birds become weaker.

On the other hand, weaker birds, reach the feeders after the stronger ones have left; they will be left with only powdery feed which they can't eat because of sharp beaks. Therefore, they also are subjected to nutrient deficiency and become weaker further.

Consequently, the entire flock shows a poor feed conversion (weight gain per kg feed consumption) and the farmer is at loss.

If the beaks are trimmed, the birds can't search for grains; instead, they have to scoop the feed and eat thereby making available all components of the feed to all the birds ensuring uniform growth, production and reproduction.

c) Avoid egg - eating vice in the layer house. Birds are very inquisitive. If by chance few eggs are broken or cracked, when the birds look at them, they peck at broken eggs. On seeing the yolk, they peck again. Once they get the taste of eggs, they start pecking at all the eggs. If the beaks are sharp, the shells may crack and the vice is stimulated. Other birds also follow and the vice spreads through the entire flock.

However, in cages, egg eating vice is not encountered because the eggs roll out of the reach of the birds soon after they are laid.

Precautions During Beak Trimming

a) How much to beak trim?

Upper beak should be trimmed 6-7 mm beyond the nostril with 2 sec of burning to block or seal blood vessels; this is referred to as "Cauterization". The lower beak should be trimmed only a few mm from the tip only to blunt its tip. In other words, upper beak is trimmed T! and the lower beak S! from the tip to nostrils.

The rule is, "Leave the Lower beak Longer", which can be remembered as "L L L Rule".

Now the question arises, why lower beak is left longer. Imagine a bird with protruding (long) upper beak. Can it eat or drink? Impossible; therefore, lower beak must be left longer than the upper beak.

b) Before beak trimming

1. Should be done during cooler hours of the day or when the temperature outside is reducing. This is to minimize the chances of bleeding, especially in the cut portion of the upper beak.
2. Administering vitamin K through drinking water 2-3 days prior to trimming can be considered as an option. Vitamin helps in blood clotting as during beak trimming, there will be bleeding especially in the upper beak.
3. Birds should not be subjected to stress from housing, vaccination or worming (medications for getting rid of worms in the intestines) during the week prior to or the week after trimming.
4. Give no medicines which will give a bad taste to the feed or water.
5. Sick birds should not be beak-trimmed.
6. Beak-trimming is not performed in combination with vaccinations (except for fowl pox) or moving of birds or medication of birds.

c) During beak-trimming

1. The operator should hold the bird in such a way that it neither shakes its head nor suffocates. If the bird shakes its head, one can't trim the beaks at all. In that anxiety, untrained operators are likely to grip the birds tightly; thus, leading to death of birds due to suffocation. In such case, the beak trimming will be successful but the bird will be dead!
2. The beaks are opened with the help of index finger and the tongue is held back. You will be scared to open the beaks; but remember, birds don't have teeth and therefore, they can't bite.
3. The upper beak is cut first to the recommended level. The beak is held against the blade and circular motion is given for at least 2 sec while holding to effect proper cauterization. Otherwise, birds start bleeding; other birds get attracted to the colour; they start pecking at the bleeding bird; cannibalism sets in.
4. Lower beak is then cut as per the recommendation.
5. Proper cauterization is once again ensured before the bird is left into the pen.

Note: If toenails have grown in excess, they can also be trimmed. Normally, if performed properly, cauterization will not be necessary.

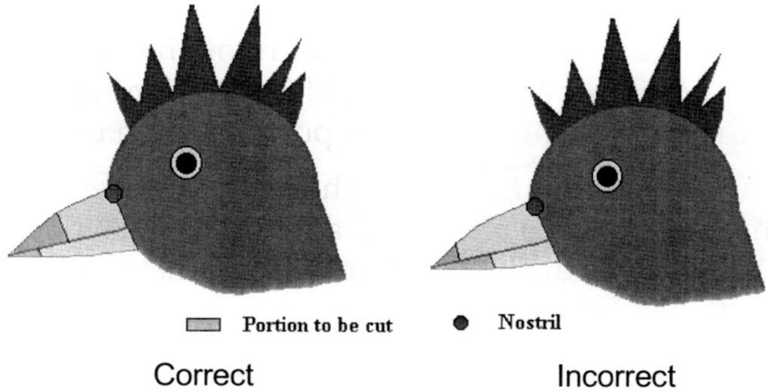

Beak trimming – procedure
(L L L rule: Leave Lower beak Longer)

d) After beak trimming

1. Feeders must be kept full with feed to help birds eat easily; probably this is the only occasion when feeders are full with feed.
2. Vitamins (B-complex and C) and vitamin K can be given through water to help reduce the stress.
3. All the birds must be observed carefully for any bleeding, especially in the upper beak. If any bird shows bleeding, it must be separated at once, suitably treated/cauterized; otherwise, there is a likelihood of cannibalism.

Caution: Adequate feed depth must be maintained in flocks with long lower beaks. Water must also be maintained at a level that will enable chickens with long lower beaks to drink without difficulty. During periods of high water consumption, it is urgent to increase the water flow so that all birds can drink regardless of their location on the water line.

Deworming

Routine (deworming) programs are relevant in the control of round worms in most management systems. However, birds in cages are not much exposed to parasite eggs and hence, under practical conditions, they are not wormed. Hence, before transfer of birds to cages from floor rearing, they are advisable to undergo worm treatment; any general worming agent (fenbendazole, mebendazole, piperazine, Ayurvedic compounds, etc.) can be used as per manufacturer's recommendations.

Most of such drugs are not palatable (not tasty); hence, birds may be deprived of water for 3 to 6 hrs (depending on weather at that time) before treatment. All drinkers are raised sufficient enough that birds can't access water. Afterwards, they are lowered down to the recommended level (level of the back of birds). Birds quickly drink the medicated water. After 24 to 48 hrs. of medication, by careful observation on the litter appearance of dead/live worms will indicate that the birds were actually had worms. In such case, vitamins, especially A and C are given for 3 days through water to help them recover faster.

Note: Same method can be practiced, whenever the given medication and or vaccine is not palatable to the birds.

Transfer of Birds to Cage Layer House

After 16 weeks of age, the pullets will be starting to produce eggs in a couple of weeks or so. Therefore, they are shifted to the Cage Layer House after 16 weeks itself so that they can get accustomed to the new rearing conditions well before they start laying eggs.

The birds are placed in crates and then shifted to cages. The birds are removed from the crates carefully and placed in cages. All through, care has to be exercised not to injure the birds; especially in the legs and or wings which are held while catching, holding, shifting and transferring.

❑❑❑

Chapter **10**

Management of Layers

The birds which now are 16 weeks old and are ready to produce eggs in about 3 or 4 weeks' time. Hence, they need a different managerial approach to make them perform to their best during the laying period. No sooner the pullet lays her first egg than she will be referred to as "Layer".

In this chapter 'Management of Layers' 17th week and onwards housed in Cage Layer House (CLH) will be discussed.

Management of Layers

During laying period also, the routine works of feeding, offering of water, healthcare and maintenance of records are continued. However, suitable changes are made for birds to be reared in cages.

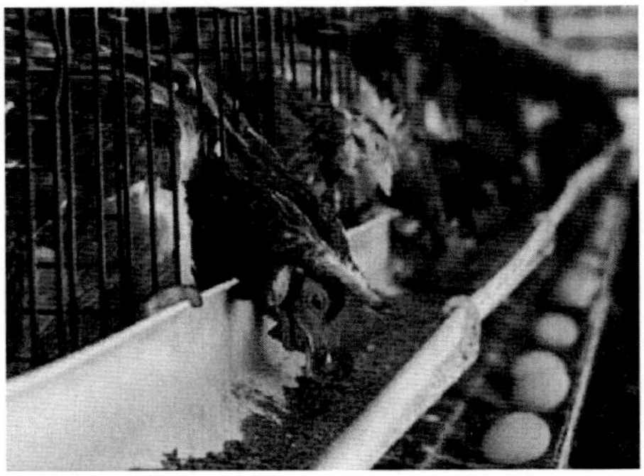

A. Manage mental recommendation for layers reared on floor

1. Living space allowances for birds on floor

The amount of space to allow will depend on climatic conditions and type of breed. However, at present all breeds are considered to be light breeds. Therefore, use the values (birds/m^2) as a guide rather than as a hard and fast rule.

Table 1: Living space allowances for layers (birds/m^2)

Age	Forced air ventilation		Natural ventilation	
	All wire floor system	Part wire floor system	All wire floor system	Art wire floor system
0-10 weeks	12	10	9	8
10-20 weeks	8	7	7	6
Laying period	8	7	7	6

Table 2: Feeder space allowances per bird on floor (Feed troughs)

1-8 weeks	16
8-16 weeks	10
16-20 weeks	12
Laying period	12

Tubular feeders

A round feeder with a pan ciramference of 50cm, equals about 100cm of trough space. When using conventional, 50 cm diameter tubular feeders provide.

Table 3: Feeder space allowances per bird (Tubular feeder)

1-18 weeks	One feeder per 35 birds
8-16 weeks	One feeder per 25 birds
16-20 weeks	One feeder per 23 birds

Table 4: Watering space per bird during different weeks

0-2 week	1 chick fountain per 100 birds
2-4 weeks	1cm/bird
4-12 weeks	2cm/bird
After 12 weeks	3cm/bird

When using round automatic drinkers, allow 1 drinker per 100 birds after 2 weeks of age.

B. Managmeental Recommendations for Layers Reared in Cages

1. Living space

   0-4 weeks: 75 birds per square meter of cage floor area

   4-20 weeks: 25 birds per square meter of cage floor area

Table 5: Stocking density of birds reared in different cages

4 deck unit system	24-27 birds/ m^2
3 deck unit system	18-20 birds / m^2
Stair step cages	10-15 birds/ m^2
Flat deck cages	12-14 birds/ m^2

Cage floor space per bird is 400 cm^2 approximately.

3. Feeder space : Allow a feeder space of 10 cm per bird.
4. Water space : One Nipple drinker is sufficient for 10 birds. A minimum of 2 Nipple drinkers per cage should be allowed.

Laying Nests

Nest boxes must be introduced to laying house two weeks prior to the onset of lay to help birds to get used to nest. The nests should be roomy, dark, cool, well-ventilated and located on one side of the shed. Clean nesting materials should be placed inside the nest boxes and the nesting material should be changed periodically.

Feeding Management

While the genetic potential of present day layer breeds for egg production has made consistent and considerable progress, simultaneously the bird's adaptability to various agro-climatic conditions, feeding practices and management practices has also improved tremendously over the last few decades. However, to optimise profits, it is necessary to provide economic but nutritionally balanced feed to obtain desired production. There are many agro-climatic zones with varying seasons and temperatures. As nutritional requirements vary from area to area and season to season, you may need to consult the local poultry nutritionist for designing feed formulation. However, in the following sections we have described general nutritional requirements. Summer makes the bird eat less and hence, efforts should be made to increase their nutritional density and bring down the temperature in the house by various means. Similarly, birds tend to eat more in winter and therefore, there is a need to make necessary changes in feed formulations. Feed consumption should also be correctly monitored so that correct nutrient levels can be provided.

Feed used in all phases of the life-cycle of poultry birds must meet the following criteria:

Nutrients should be supplied in proper proportions and in a form which is bio-available to the birds.

- Texture, colour, taste of feed must be acceptable to the birds.
- Feed must not be dusty.

Ideally feed must be free from following contaminants:

- All pathogenic organisms
- Harmful chemicals and
- Toxins

If animal by-products like meat-meal, fish-meal, liver-meal, blood-meal and hydrolysed feather-meal are used, care should be taken to ensure that they are free from all types of contaminants. Soyabean meal, used in poultry feed, must have been properly roasted. Inadequate or excess heat during processing of soyabean for oil extraction will damage the nutritional value of soyabean. The level of roasting of soybean can be judged by feed analytical laboratories.

Calcium should be added to the feed in form of oyster-shell with particle size of 2.5 mm to 3.5 mm. If calcium is to be added in the form of limestone, 2/3rd should be used as large particles (3-5 mm) and only 1/3rd in the form of powder. Limestone so used, should be low in magnesium.

Contamination of feed during storage, transport and delivery must be avoided. Wild-birds and rodents can contaminate the feed in any of the above stages.

If you are making your own feed, formulate your feed according to the season, age & body weight and production level of the birds. The formulations should be based on the actual weight of different ingredients and the accurate valuation of each feed ingredient before they are added together.

Feeding Recommendations for commercial layers

- Chick Mash : Chick mash should be fed to the birds from its arrival until the average body weight of the birds reaches 580 g. This is a feed-to-weight program rather than feed-to-age program. Body weight gains are better with pelleted/crumbled feed compared to mash feed. Therefore, it is recommended to use pelleted/crumbled chick feed.
- Grower Mash : The grower feed should be fed till flock reaches an average body weight of 1100 g. Do not administer pre-lay feed to the birds weighing below 1100 g.
- Pre-lay Feed : Care should be taken to ensure pre-lay feed is introduced after the flock attains an average body weight of 1100 g and usually for two to three weeks.
- Layer Feed : Layer feed offered to the laying birds should be formulated according to the age of the birds and egg production. Accordingly, layer feed can be divided into three groups i.e. Phase I, Phase II and Phase III. Phase I feed should be given upto the age of 40 weeks and later Phase II ration may be given. Phase III feed should be given after the age of 60 weeks. Phase feeding saves money.

Table 6: Suggested Nutritional Requirements Pre- lay and Laying Period

	Pre-lay Feed	**Phase I**	**Phase II**	**Phase III**
Age in weeks	16 to 18	19 to 40	41 to 60	61 onwards
Metabolizable Energy kcal/kg	2500	2500	2500	2500
Crude Protein % (min.)	17.0	17.5	16.0	15.5
Methionine % (min.)	0.40	0.40	0.30	0.30
Lysine % (min.)	0.72	0.80	0.70	0.70
Calcium % (min)	2.50	3.60	4.00	4.00
Available Phosphorous % (min.)	0.40	0.35	0.30	0.30

Table 7: Feed Consumption and Body Weight target of commercial layers (Growing Phase)

Age		Grams of Feed per Bird		Body Weight in g
Weeks	Days	Per Day	Cumulative	
1	0 - 7	11	77	70
2	8 - 14	16	189	120
3	15 - 21	18	315	170
4	22 - 28	25	490	230
5	29 - 35	35	735	310
6	36 - 42	40	1015	410
7	43 - 49	44	1323	490
8	50 - 56	48	1659	580
9	57 - 63	49	2002	640
10	64 - 70	50	2352	740
11	71 - 77	51	2709	820
12	78 - 84	54	3087	900
13	85 - 91	56	3479	970
14	92 - 98	58	3885	1030
15	99 - 105	60	4305	1070
16	106 - 112	62	4739	1110
17	113 - 119	63	5180	1160
18	120 - 126	66	5642	1200
19	127 - 133	75	6167	1280
20	134 - 140	82	6741	1360

Light Requirement

Light entering the eyes of birds induces response in the hypothalamus which through releasing factors in turn affects the rate of secretion of gonado tropic hormones, which affects the activity of the gonads and in turn the reproductive behaviour of birds. Age of sexual maturity and rate of egg production are affected by pattern of lighting in laying house but this does not have the power either to stop and start these reproductive processes. If natural light is short at the time of laying, the light period should be increased gradually by providing weekly increments of 15 minutes upto maximum of 16 hours.

A. Windowless houses

There should be even distribution of light. Suspend the bulbs 2 meters above the floor level. Allow 60-walts per bird per 15 sq m of floor area.

Table 8: Light intensity for layer chicken

0-2 weeks	4 walts per sq. Mts
2-4 weeks	3 walts per sq. Mts
4-20 weeks	2 walts per sq. Mts
Laying period	3.2 walts per sq. Mt

With florescent light, use 25% of the given walts/ m^2. Never increase light intensity not even for a short time.

Duration of light

Never increase day-length during the rearing period and never reduce day-length during the laying period. If the flock fails to come into lay at a sufficiently rapid rate, increasing total light at 24 weeks upto 15 hours may help to stimulate the production.

B. Conventional Houses

A separate lighting schedule for windowless houses can be adopted for the layers.

Provide whenever possible

- An 8 hours day (natural and artificial) at 20 weeks of age.
- A 14 hours day (natural and artificial) at 23 weeks of age.
- Increase every two weeks day length by 30 minutes upto a maximum of 18 hours, once 80% rate of lay is reached but not later than 32 weeks of age.
- Set the morning lights to burn until a little after sunrise. In addition, set the clock so that evening lights turn on before dusk.
- On dark days, the light should be on all day. Provide a minimum light intensity in the laying period of 3.2 watts/sq.mt.
- Use both artificial morning and evening lights. This will help to maintain a more constant-day-length.

- The step-down programme can be practised as follows:
  a) Take the natural day-length at 20 weeks of age of the flock.
  b) Add to the day-length 6 hours. That gives artificial day-length at 6 weeks.
  c) For day-length before 6 weeks follow the basic schedule for houses without windows till the point the necessary day length of 6 weeks is reached.

Light is the most important stimulant for egg production. Hence, special care is essential as far as lighting management in a CLH.

Type of bulbs

Incandescent bulbs with flat reflectors are preferred for poultry houses Incandescent light contain more red colour; red colour is a better stimulant for egg production. Further, fluorescent light is efficient only when the temperature is around the ideal 21.1°C (70°F).This is because the birds are in cages located below the light source. Therefore, there is no need of illuminating the roof of the house; instead, it can be reflected downwards so that wattage can be reduced; in turn, power (electricity) consumption can be reduced. Why flat reflectors are required? This is because the round reflectors create round areas of light and between bulbs, triangular areas of darkness is produced. On the contrary, with the flat reflectors, the entire area is illuminated.Usually, 40 or 60 W incandescent bulbs are used in CLH.

Fixing of bulb and reflector

Bulbs are fixed above the passages only. This is because light is required so that the feed and nipple drinkers are visible and to stimulate egg production through the eyes. If the bulbs are fixed over the cages, only shadow of the cages fall on the birds (eyes).

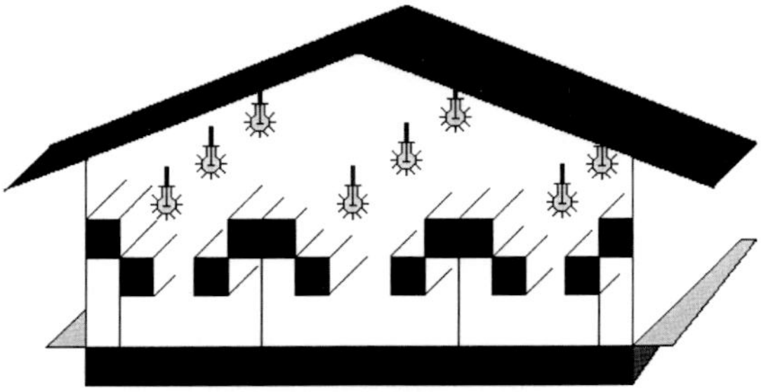

Arrangement of bulbs in a CLH

Bulb and reflector are fixed straight from the roof. The bulbs are fixed in such a way that distance between two bulbs in a row is 1½ times the height at which the bulbs are fixed. Bulbs are generally fixed at a height of 2.1 to 2.4 m (7 to 8 ft) height so that it will not obstruct men working inside. Therefore, the distance between two bulbs must be 3.15 to 3.60 m (10.5 to 12.0 ft).

Each of the bulb-reflector assembly is fixed straight from the roof. If the bulbs are loose, the assembly will move due to winds or some other reason. It will make the shadows also to move which is likely to frighten the birds resulting in reduced egg production.

Cleaning of bulbs and reflectors

Cleanliness of the bulb and reflector is also important and clean reflectors, on most occasions, improve the light efficiency by about 50% since they reflect the light that would have been absorbed by the ceiling. Therefore, both bulb and reflectors must be cleaned once a fortnight or more frequently.

Duration of light (Photoperiod)

The total duration of light, including sunlight is referred to as "Photoperiod". A photoperiod of 15½ to 16 hrs. is recommended. A sudden change in duration of light and/or feed should not be done and only a gradual change must be made in length of the light day (photoperiod). When the first eggs are laid (about 20 weeks of age), it is advisable to consider the change of lighting program. The additional light other than the natural daylight may be given either before the sunrise or after sunset or a combination of both; the latter is more convenient, as it coincides with normal working schedule. That means 4 am to 6 am and 6 pm to 8 pm. Many farmers install a timer to put on and off the lights at the desired timings. Hence, under commercial conditions, duration of light is increased by ½ hr per week (from 20th week) till a maximum of 16-17 hr is attained and maintained at that from then onwards.

A question normally arises; why not 24 hrs. light. Layers must never be given continuous (24 hr) light; excess light results in excess feed consumption, fat accumulation, hyperexcitation, cannibalism, prolapse, reduced egg production, etc.

Culling for Production

The most accurate method of measuring a birds productive ability is by trap nesting record. However, only a small fraction of the total population can be culled by this method. Therefore, out of a practical necessity, birds have to be culled by external appearance. A successful poultry farmer practices year round culling in conformity with his handling and other managemental practices to obtain maximum advantages.

Culling Birds for Present Production

Laying flocks are generally to be liquidated after one year of production since keeping them longer into the second year of production may be uneconomical.

Year round culling of unproductive stock will fetch better profit. Culling is based on morphological factors or characters which reflect physiological changes related to production. However, a bird must be in good physical condition in order to enable one to judge its production satisfactorily.

To judge whether a bird is laying or not, the following characters associated with hen's performance are examined:

1. The vent of a laying hen is large, moist and dilated and tends to be oblong in shape. The lower edge appears flat and extends almost straight across and the upper edge blends evenly into the surrounding tissues, which have a smooth loose, pliable appearance. In contrast to this, the vent of a non-laying hen is small, contracted and dry. The region-around the vent is puckered, round and hard.
2. The pubic bones of a lying hen are wide, apart, usually the width of two or more fingers in comparison with the rather close-fitting (one or two fingers width) pubic bones of the non-producer. Moreover, pubic bones of a lying hen are thin and pliable in contrast to rigid pubics of a non-laying hen.
3. In a producing hen, the comb wattles and ear lobes usually appear large, smooth, red and waxy.

These characteristics are prominent, when the pullet comes into the height of her production. As the laying season advances, these head appendages lose their gloss and towards the end of production become dull or pale in colour and reduced in size. The comb of a bird which is out of production is small, contracted, dry and cool to touch. The comb being very prominent by visible, provides one of the best and easily discernible external characteristics, which can indicate a non-producing hen in a poultry farm.

Table 9: Characters for judging present Production

Character	Layer	Non-layer
1. Vent	Large, dilated, oblong, moist	Small. Contracted, round, dry
2. Pubic bones	Wide apart (usually 3 fingers width)	Close together (one or two fingers width)
3. Comb	Large, red, full, glossy, warm	Small, pale, scaly, cold
4. Wattles and ear lobes	Prominent, soft, smooth	Icons copious, rough, dry
5. Admiral capacity	A depth of 4-5 fingers from the end of keel to the pubic bones	A depth of 2-3 fingers only
6. Handling	a) Soft and pliable abdomen b) Pubic bones, thin, pliable c) Low substanoues fat	a) Abdomen not flexible and rubbery b) Rigid c) High

Culling for intensity of Production

Intensity may be defined as the rate of egg production i.e. the number of eggs laid per unit of time. It is controlled by clutch size and the interval length. The eggs laid on consecutive days i.e. without interruption is referred to as a clutch and the number of eggs laid in each clutch determines the clutch size. An average clutch size of floor or more eggs is essential towards making a high annual egg record. The interval of length is the time in hours between successive eggs. The two physical characters which seem to be more, closely associated with intensity are abdominal capacity and handling quality.

1. Abdominal capacity

Abdominal capacity may be determined by measuring the distance between the keel and the pubic bones. The ovary and oviduct of a hen in full production are enlarges (about 20 times) than in a dormant condition. Besides, due to increased appetite and enlargement, digestive organs require more space in the body cavity, which in part is brought about by a dropping or lowering of the keel. A depth of

4-5 fingers from the end of the keel to the pubic bone indicates good capacity, while a depth of 2-3 fingers indicates fair to poor capacity.

2. Handling quality

Handling quality refers to the physical condition of a pullet, when she reaches sexual maturity. An intense layer always draws on its reserve fat as the laying season progresses which cause changes in certain regions of the body of the hen, reflecting its intensity of production. Good layers show the following changes:

a) Abdomen becomes soft and pliable in contrast to non-flexible or rubbery abdomen of the low intensity bird.

b) The pubic bones become thin and pliable in contrast to the rigid well-cushioned bones of the low rate hen.

c) The shanks became flattened, instead of nbeing round as in the low rate hen.

d) Subcutaneous fat is practically absent in birds of high intensity.

Culling for persistency of production

Persistency is the ability of the hen to lay eggs well, even towards the end of her laying year. It has the same effect at the end of the laying year, as early maturity does at all beginning. Persistency can be judged either by trap nest records or from certain changes in physical characters. The two characters that are associated with persistency of egg production are pigmentation and moult:

1. **Pigmentation :** The presence of pigments in certain regions of the body of hen and their bleaching is in itself of great value in predicting the length of time; the birds have been in production. However, unfortunately, it is limited to only those breeds that have yellow skin. Plymouth Rocks, Rhode Islands, Leghorns and Hampshire have characteristic while Orpington has white skin. Minorca has black shanks so pigmentation is of no value in culling these birds. The yellow colour is due to the pigment Xanthophylls, which is derived from feed stuffs like yellow maize and green feeds. In non-laying birds, the yellow pigments are deposited in the skin and the fatty tissues underlying the skin, when production starts, the Xanthophyll of feed is diverted directly from the intestinal wall into the developing ova or yolk instead

of being distributed into the fatty tissues of the body. Since the source of supply is diverted, the yellow pigment of the body is gradually bleached due to oxidation process. This disappearance of the pigment from the body tissues is called bleaching.

It requires 20-24 weeks of production for all of these regions to be completely bleached. Fading out of pigments is of considerable value in estimating the length of the time a bird has been in production up to 6 months. Thereafter, it is considered in conjunction with moult which gives best results. When a bird stops laying the reappearance or return of pigments, follows the same order in which they have disappeared but is more rapid. Bleaching takes place in a regular order.

Table 10: Order of bleaching from the different regions of the body

S.No.	Region bleached	No. of weeks in production
1.	Vent	1-2 weeks
2.	Eye ring	
3.	Ear lobes	2-4 weeks
4.	Base of beak	
5.	Tip of beak	6-8 weeks
6.	Bottom of feet	8-10 weeks
7.	Front of shanks	
8.	Rear of shanks	20-24 weeks
9.	Hock joint	

2. **Moulting :** The shedding and renewal of feathers is referred to as moulting which occurs once in a year, though it may occur twice during the same period in some birds. The order in which feathers of different sections of the body are lost is rather definite. The usual order is head, neck, body (including breast, back, and abdomen) wings and tail. When the moult extends to the body and wings, the hens usually stop laying and the moult becomes complete.

The primary feathers (which are 10 in number) are the stiff flight feathers seen on the outer part of the wing, when it is spread out. These are separated from the secondary feathers (1-4 in number) by a short feather, known as the axial feather. The primary feathers are moulted from the axial feathers towards the tip of the wing in succession until the lost one to be dropped is the outer most primary feather. The secondary's which moult after the primaries; do not follow such a regular order. It takes about 6 weeks for a new feather to grow out both in low and high producers, but the latter grows more feathers at a time thereby completing the moult much more quickly than a low producer.

An early moulter replaces the primary feathers singly or not more than two at a time. Hens postponing the moult till late in the laying season moult rapidly dropping three or more feathers at a time, which requires a six week period to mature i.e., the same duration is required by a single primary feather. Not only this, but best producers continue to lay during a part or all the time a wing moult is in progress. Occasionally, a hen amay even, replaces only a part of the primaries while retaining the remaining feathers for the second year of the lay.

Table 11: Difference between High producers and Low producers

S.No.	High producers	Low producers
1.	Continue to lay well and moult very late towards the end of the layer year	Get into moult early during the year
2.	Are fast moulters, shed 3 or more feathers at a time	Are slow moulters, shed only one feather at a time
3.	Grow more number of new feathers at a time	Grow only one feather at a time.
4.	Complete the moult in s hort time	Take considerably long time to complete moult
5.	Continue to lay while moulting	Stop laying early
6.	Come back into production early	Take long time to come back into laying

Culling for combines characters (Intensity and Persistency)

The two important characters, intensity and persistency can be applied together in culling the birds. However, on difficulty in placing birds correctly is that a bird may be persistent but lay at a higher rate but lack persistency

Egg Producing ability Intensity	(Body capacity and Handling quality)
	Persistency (Pigmentation and moult)

❑❑❑

Chapter **11**

Feeding of Poultry

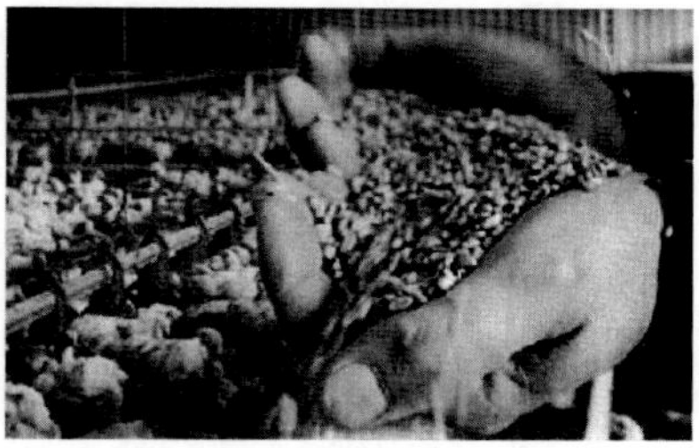

Feed cost alone constitutes about 65-70% of total cost of production of poultry meat and eggs. Scientific and balanced feeding of poultry is of primary importance to ensure high and continuous production. Since major expenditure in poultry raising is feed cost, economic consideration assumes a vital significance. In the final analysis, efficient ration with minimum cost appear to be the principal need of the poultry man. The major nutrient required by poultry is water, protein, carbohydrates, fat, minerals and vitamins. The carbohydrate and fat are the principal energy sources. Fat are the concentrated form of energy and yield 2.25 times more energy than carbohydrate on the basis of weight. Protein is essentially required to meet the requirement of amino acids. Some of these called non-essential amino acids are synthesized in the body. Hence, must be supplied through the diet. Minerals and vitamin do not supply energy but regulate several metabolic processes in the body. A balanced ration is the one which will supply different nutrients in right proportions according to the requirements for maintenance and various productive functions. The nutrients required by poultry must be supplied in rations through the ingredients available in sufficient quantity economically. Feeding to growing and productive poultry is an important work that is carried out daily at regular interval by trained supporting staff of the poultry farm. Two types of poultry feed are prepared. One is ready-made and in the form of mash or pellets. The second is in concentrated form for mixing with an energy source. Concentrates are protein sources, balanced in amino acids and containing vitamins, minerals and feed additives. They are mixed with energy sources, such as maize, sorghum or bajra to prepare poultry rations.

- **Digestive System in Chicken**: The functions of digestive system of chicken are given below:
- **Mouth:** Birds feed through the beak. The horny upper and lower mandibles form the beak. Lips, teeth, cheek and soft palate are absent. The dagger like tongue helps to force the feed into the oesophagus.
- **Oesophagus:** It is made of loose fibrous tissue and serves as a tube to pass the food from mouth to crop.
- **Crop:** It is a pouch like structure of oesophagus to store, moisten and soften the food.
- **Proventriculus or Glandular stomach or True stomach:** It is an enlarged glandular ovoid structure of the oesophagus connected to gizzard. It secretes Pepsin and Hydrochloric acid.
- **Gizzard or muscular stomach:** Disc shaped muscular organ with two pairs of strong thick muscles and lined internally with a thick horny epithelial covering called the *Koilin* layer. Coarse materials are ground well by its powerful contractions with support of the grit that bird consumes.
- **Small Intestines:** It comprises of duodenum, jejunum and ileum. It is the site of digestion and absorption. The duodenal loop supports the pancreas that secretes pancreatic juice. In chicken, the absorption regions of the small intestine have a capillary bed instead of central lacteals of the villi.
- **Caeca:** Two blind ended pouch-like structure that demarcates the small and large intestines. Here, microbial digestion of the undigested food material takes place.
- **Large intestine:** This part of gut is very small and the size is doubled the diameter of small intestine with a short rectum. This is the site of water absorption.
- **Cloaca**: This is a bulb like structure at the end of the digestive tract that serves as the common exit for digestive, reproductive and urinary tracts. Faeces are urine pass out simultaneously as a brownish black mass with whitish uric acid cap on its top.
- **Vent:** This is the external opening of the cloaca.
- **Supplementary digestive organs:** The supplementary digestive organs assist the digestive process are the pancreas and liver.

- **Pancreas:** It secretes the pancreatic juice that is conveyed into the duodenum through the pancreatic duct. The pancreatic enzymes digest the carbohydrates, proteins and fats.
- **Liver:** It secretes greenish yellowish sticky bile that helps to emulsify the fat for digestion and to neutralize the acidic condition of the digestive tract.

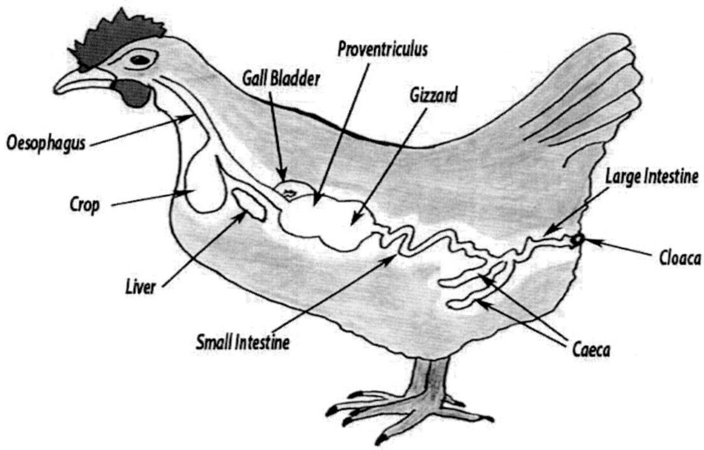

Digestive System of Chicken

Feeding of poultry

Proper nutrition of poultry is important for the following reasons:

a) Poor quality food is not digested easily and causes ill health, lower vitality, retards growth and development and also reduces egg production.

b) Intensive system of raising poultry demands proper feed mixtures.

d) The relative feed cost of different feeds their feed value availability needs special attention in formulating proper feed mixtures.

c) Increased flock size.

d) Use of agricultural by-products in feed.

e) Preparation of feeds for specific purpose and for economic and efficient production.

Purpose of poultry feeding

1. To transfer inedible or less edible products into edible or highly delicious or nutritious food like meat and egg.

2. To meet the physiological needs of the bird, such as:
   a) Maintenance
   b) Heat to produce body temperature
   c) Energy for action
   d) Growth
   e) Reproduction
   f) Fattening

Principles of poultry feeding

1. Birds have no lips and teeth and hence, cannot chew the feeds therefore, ration must have mainly concentrates (grains, oil cake, by products).
2. Birds have simple stomach, hence requirements are more precise and specific.
3. Birds have higher rate of metabolism than other farm animals, therefore different feed for different class of birds is required as per recommended standards.
4. They are fed in groups.
5. Birds have no sweat glands to cool down their body, hence their respiration, pulse rate and body temperature is relatively higher. Consequently their metabolic rate is higher. Accordingly, nutritional adjustments are needed.
6. Feed must be free from Aflatoxins.
7. Clean, fresh and cool water must be made available at all times.
8. Birds are non-ruminants and hence, feed must contain not more than 6 to 7 per cent of crude fibre.
9. Birds are reared for different purpose (meat, egg, etc.) and hence, according to purpose, age, breed, size and system of rearing the requirements must be determined with definite ratio of protein and energy.
10. Feed must have all essential nutrients in balanced form.

Table 1: BIS Specification of poultry feed, 1992 (Feeding standard)

Characteristics	Broiler Pre-starter	Broiler starter	Broiler finisher	Chick	Grower	Layer	Breeder
Moisture % by wt (max)	11	11	11	11	11	11	11
Crude protein %	23	22	20	20	16	18	18
Crude fibre % by wt (max)	6	6	6	7	8	8	8
Acid insoluble ash % by wt (max)	3	3	3	4	4	4	4
Salt % by wt (max)	0.6	0.6	0.6	0.6	0.6	0.6	0.6
Calcium % by wt (min)	1.2	1.2	1.2	1.0	1.0	3.0	3.0
Phosphorus % by wt (min)	0.5	0.5	0.5	0.5	0.5	0.5	0.5
Lysine % by wt (min)	1.2	1.2	1.0	0.9	0.6	0.65	0.65
DL-Methionine % by wt (min)	0.65	0.50	0.35	0.30	0.25	0.30	0.30
Metabolizable energy Kcal/kg min	2800	2900	3000	2600	2500	2600	2600
Manganese mg/kg	90	90	50	55	90	90	90
Iodine mg/kg	1	1	1	1	1	1	1
Iron mg/kg	120	120	90	75	120	120	90
Copper mg/kg	15	12	9	9	12	12	-
Vitamin A IU/kg	6000	6000	6000	8000	6000	6000	8000
Vitamin D3 IU/kg	600	600	600	1200	600	600	1200
Thiamine mg/kg	6	5	3	5	5	3	-
Riboflavin mg/kg	6	6	5	5	6	6	8
Pantothenic acid mg/kg	15	15	15	5	15	15	15
Nicotinic acid mg/kg	40	40	15	15	40	40	15
Biotin mg/kg	0.3	0.3	0.15	0.15	0.3	0.3	0.15
Vitamin B12 mg/kg	0.015	0.015	0.010	0.010	0.015	0.010	-
Zinc mg/kg	50	50	75	60	60	100	-

Table 2: Feed requirement for poultry

Age	Feed (gm) per bird
1st week	10-15
2-3rd week	30-50
4-8th week	60-70
8-20th week	70-90
20 week onwards	110

Table 3: Water requirement for poultry

Age	Water requirement per 100 birds/ day (Liters)
1-3 week	2-6
3-6 week	7-14
6-10 week	15-20
10-17 week	20-25
18-20 week onwards	25-30
Laying hens	30-35

Proximate Composition of Poultry

Feed is the largest component of expenditure, which accounts for more than 75% of poultry production.

Nutrient requirements are known more precisely for poultry than other species of animal. Proper poultry ration can be devised only by the application of the nutritional information about the class of poultry to be fed. This requires knowledge of the nutrients, the feed stuffs available to supply these nutrients and the amount of nutrient needed for the particular purpose.

Nutrients are essential substances that are present in feeds. These are required for growth, maintenance and reproductive process of a living body. Poultry require more than 40 such nutrients, which are classified into six major groups based on their chemical nature, their functions and the method of determination.

These are: 1. Proteins 2. Carbohydrates. 3. Fats. 4. Minerals 5, Vitamins and 6. Water.

1. Proteins

Proteins were so named because these substances are of primary importance to the body, as they perform innumerable vital functions. (The word "**Protein**" is of Greek origin. "**Proto**" in Greek means **first** or **primary**) Enzymes, hormones and antibodies are all proteins.

Proteins are first broken down to their basic units "amino acids" in the digestive tract by the enzymes and then absorbed. In the chicken body, proteins are the major constituents of the structural and protective tissues, such as skin, feathers, bones, muscles, ligaments and organs. They are also important for growth and egg production.

The absolutely essential amino acids for chicken include arginine, histidine, isoleucine, leucine, lysine, methionine, phenylaline, threonine, trytophane and valine. Of these, methionine and lysine are the most critical amino acids that should be taken into account while formulating ration for poultry. Both plant sources of protein (Soyabean meal, groundnut extract, sunflower meal), and animal sources of protein (fish meal, meat meal, bone meal) are used in poultry feed.

2. Carbohydrates

Carbohydrates are the major sources of energy and heat for the body. They are required for maintenance of body temperature, growth, bird activity and production activity and production of eggs. Excess carbohydrates in the body are converted into fats. The major ingredients that contribute carbohydrates in poultry feed are the cereals and grains, such as maize, wheat, jowar, rice, etc.

3. Fats

Fats are another potential major source of energy. They supply essential fatty acids like linoleic acids and arachidonic acid. Fats are the most concentrated source of energy that a bird can consume. They have a gross energy value of 9.45 Kcal compared to only 4.1 Kcal for a typical carbohydrates. They are digested and metabolized with high efficiency . Fats are the only components, which are deposited intact into tissues with little or no modification. Because of their high energy content, relatively large amounts of fats or oils are added to some poultry rations, particularly in broiler diets.

Fats are important components of vital lipid known as **"Phospholipids".** They are found in all living cells and in the cell (plasma) membrane. Both linoleic acid and arachidonic are important constituents of phospholipids. Linoleic acid cannot be synthesized in the chicken body but can be converted to arachidonic acid. Essential fatty acid deficiency in laying hens results in low egg production, egg size and hatchability. Most commercial feed ingredients are low in linoleic acid. Linoleic acid is required for maintaining satisfactory egg size and weight.

The fat content of the nervous tissue is also high. Fat also serves as an insulating material in the subcutaneous tissue of the skin and around certain organs.

4. Vitamins

Vitamins are a group of organic substances that are essential in minute quantities for normal growth of the bird, maintenance, and egg production. Since they are vital for life and all contain the amino group (NH_2) in their structure, they are called "Vitamin".(In Latin "Vita" means life. Vita+ amino= vital amine, or "Vitamin"). Vitamins are neither sources of energy nor do they serve as building blocks. But they are effective in minute quantities. They act mainly as regulators of metabolic processes and play a role in energy transformations, usually acting as co-enzymes in enzymatic systems.

Vitamins exist in most foods in minute amounts in their natural state. All vitamins, except vitamin C, are essential for poultry. Although the amounts of vitamins required in poultry diets range from parts per million (ppm) to parts per billion (ppb), each is required for normal metabolism and health. A marked deficiency of a single vitamin in the diet of chick leads to breakdown of the metabolic process in which that particular vitamin is involved. This results in a vitamin deficiency disease.

There are 13 vitamins necessary for the chicken.

Vitamins are classified into two groups:

1. Fat-soluble vitamins – – – – Vitamin A, D, E and K
2. Water-soluble vitamins – – – Vitamin B group and Vitamin C.

5. Minerals

Besides carbohydrates, fats, proteins and vitamins, many other elements form a part of the bird's nutritional requirements. These are essential "mineral elements". Minerals are as important as amino acids and vitamins in the maintenance of life, well-being, and production in poultry. They enter into composition of bones and give the skeletal the rigidity and strength needed to support the soft tissues. Minerals combine with proteins, lipids and other substances that make up the soft tissues. Minerals are also necessary for activation of many enzymes of the body. In most cases, the necessary quantity required for each is very small.

At least 13 minerals are required for the best health and productivity of birds. Minerals that perform structural or osmotic functions are required in relatively large amounts in the diet and are referred to as "macro-mineral":

Calcium	Phosphorus
Sodium	Potassium
Chlorine	Magnesium

Minerals that are required in relatively low amount in the diet are referred to as "Micro-minerals", "Trace elements". These include:

Copper	Iodine
Iron	Manganese
Selenium	Zinc

All the above macro-minerals and trace minerals are essential for the well-being of birds. Fluorine in small amounts is a constant constituent of several tissues, particularly bones. Analysis of each mineral in the body of chicken has revealed that major portions of calcium, phosphorus, magnesium and zinc are present in bones. Other essential elements are distributed largely in muscles, other soft tissues, and body fluids.

Classification of Common feed Ingredients for Poultry

Conveniently, poultry feed ingredients can be widely classified into:

- Energy sources: Maize, rice polish, wheat bran, de-oiled rice bran, sorghum, molasses, fats and oils.
- Proteinaceous (animal origin): Fish meal, meat meal, slaughter house by product meal, hydrolysable poultry feather meal, hatchery by-product meal and silkworm pupae meal.
- Proteinaceous (plant origin): Soyabean meal, groundnut cake, cottonseed cake, sesame cake and canola meal.
- Mineral supplement: Dicalcium phosphate, Limestone and oyster shell.

The type of feed ingredients used in conventional poultry rations usually depends on their availability. Cereals like maize, rice, wheat, oat, barley; cereal by products, such as wheat bran or rice polish; and animal and vegetable protein sources like fish meal, soybean oil meal and groundnut cake. The whole ration is fortified with adequate amount of minerals and vitamins. With the cost of feed soaring high and the availability of conventional ingredients becoming scarce, intensive and continuous efforts are being made to determine the nutritive value of agro- industrial by-products to replace most costly ingredients in rations. The following are some of the feed stuffs used for making poultry rations:

Energy sources

- Maize : This is a widely used poultry feed ingredient. It is highly digestible and contains little fibre. It is used as a source of energy and is low in protein, especially lysine and sulphur containing amino acids. The yellow varieties are good source of vitamin A and xanthophylls. The latter is responsible for the yellow skin in certain breeds of fowl. This will improve the yolk colour.
- Barley: Barley is not very palatable because of its high fibre content and should not constitute more than 15% of the ration.
- Oat: It should not constitute more than 20% of the ration. Manganese content in it helps in preventing hock disorder, feather pulling and cannibalism.
- Wheat: Wheat can replace as a source of energy, but it is very costly.
- Wheat bran: It is bulky and quite laxative on account of its high fibre manganese and phosphorus content.

- Bajra: This is very useful feedstuff and is similar to wheat in its nutritive value.
- Rice: Broken grains of rice can be used for feeding.
- Rice polish: This is a very good substitute for cereal grains. It can be used upto 50 per cent of the ration. Because of the high oil content, it often becomes rancid on storage.
- De-oiled rice polish: Energy content of de-oiled rice polish is low because of the removal of fat, but it is rich in protein and ash content. Its feeding value is lower than that of the regular rice polish.
- Rice bran: It is used as energy source. Because of high fibre content, it can be used only upto 15-20%.
- Sorghum: Its feeding value is similar to that of maize, but has higher protein content. It is quite palatable. Sorghum-meal is a good source of some amino acids.
- Tapioca meal:. Certain varieties contain cyanogenic substances which can be removed during processing of tapioca by sun drying or heating.
- Hominy feed: It is the by-product obtained during dry milling of maize. This consists of bran germ and part of starchy part of kernels. It resembles maize in composition but is less used due to its high fibre content and lower energy value.
- Dried poultry waste: It is high in calcium and phosphorus and contains about 10-12% true protein. If treated properly, it can be included in the diet up to 10% without any detrimental effect.
- Fats: Many animal and vegetable fats are used for formulating high energy starter and broiler rations. These include beef tallow, lard mutton fat and many other edible oils. Usually 3-8% is included in the ration. However, the cost of such inclusions vis-a-vis returns should be considered. Since fats are prone to oxidative rancidity, addition of 0.02% antioxidant to the rations will counter cat rancidity.

Protein sources

The protein sources may be classified into those of animal and plant origin. The usefulness of protein feeds depend on their digestibility and the potential to furnish the essential amino acids required by the bird for body growth and production. As a general rule, use of two or three protein feedstuffs provides a better assortment of amino acids and other nutrients than a single once.

Vegetable Protein Sources

Groundnut cake

It is quite palatable and is widely used as a source of protein. It contains about 40% protein.

Mustard cake

It is superior to groundnut cake in protein quality and lysine content. However, its use in poultry ration is limited because of glycosides and goitrogens. Even if treated or processed, its use should be limited to 5 per cent in chick and not over 10 per cent in layer diets.

Soyabean meal

Soybean meals contains about 35-40 per cent protein and 18-21 per cent fat. A suitable heat treatment improves protein quality of the meal. Soyabean contain good amount of all essential amino acids.

Sesame meal

It contains about 38 per cent protein and can be used in poultry rations.

Sunflower meal

It is superior to groundnut meal in its nutritive value. High fibre content restricts its use in poultry ration.

Cottonseed cake

It is rich in protein content but deficient in lysine. It can substitute groundnut cake upto 15% only. Continuous use of this cake in layers causes yolk mottling on storage of eggs due to gossypol content.

Linseed meal

It is a good source of tryptophan. The meals contain the toxic principles cyanogenic glucosids and antipyridoxil factor and can not be used more than 5 per cent, if not processed. The meal can be rendered non-toxic by boiling.

Maize gluten meal

These are by-products of starch industry and are rich in protein and provitamin A and xanthophylls.

Animal protein sources

Fish meal

Fish meal is one of the best poultry feed stuffs as a source of protein. Most fish meals contain 45-55% protein. The presence of fish scales reduces its feeding value.

Blood meal

Blood collected at slaughter houses is coagulated and dried to produce the meal. Blood meal contains 80 per cent protein. It can be included up to 2-3 per cent due to unpalatability and low biological value of its protein.

Meat meal

It is usually a slaughter house by-product and is prepared by curing and drying the carcass wastes. It contains 55-65% crude protein content. It can replace fish meal fully in the chick rations. It can be included at 5-10 per cent in all poultry rations.

Liver residue meal

It is a by-product of pharmaceutical industry. It can replace all fish meal.

Hatchery by-product meal

This consists of infertile eggs, dead embryos; killed chicks and egg shells collected as wastes during hatchery operations, and have been cooked dried and ground with or without removal of part or its fat. It contains 25-34 per cent protein depending upon its ingredients.

Feather meal

It contains 80-85 per cent of crude protein and may be used up to 5 per cent level in various poultry rations.

Poultry by-product meal

This product is from poultry processing plants. It includes heads, feet, etc. It contains 55-60 per cent protein.

Bone meal

It is a good source of high quality protein, calcium and phosphorus. This can be included in Poultry feeds at 5-10 per cent level.

Feed Additive

A feed additive or supplement is a substance or mixture of substances, other than the bulk and basic feedstuffs, used in small quantities, usually at less than one per cent level in the compounded feeds, in order to supplement and complement certain nutrients or non-nutrients to improve the quality of the feed and performance of birds fed.

Functions of Feed additives

Feed additives have one or more of the following functions:

- Prevent various deficiency diseases mostly nutritional origin diseases.
- Improve the nutritive value of the feed and feed efficiency.
- Improve the growth rate and egg production.
- Protect the birds from stress and improve the immune status.
- Prevent the spoilage of feed due to microbes, rancidity and other physical conditions.
- Enhance the colour, flavour, palatability and general appearance of the feed.
- Help to prevent caking, dustiness and loss of feed during storage and handling and feeding.
- Improve the quality of the egg, yolk colour, shell thickness and meat quality.
- Have sparing action on certain nutrients and prevent nutritional imbalance, facilitate better absorption of nutrients.
- Certain non-nutrient feed additives cause thinning of gut wall and thereby facilitate better absorption of nutrients.

Based on their functions, the feed additives are broadly classified into two categories as:

a) Nutrient feed additives.

b) Non-nutrient feed additives.

c) Nutrient feed additives.

The nutrient feed additives contain essential nutrients necessary for normal growth and production of the birds. Deficiency of these in poultry will lead to various anatomical and physiological abnormalities. The nutrient feed additives can be categorized.

1. Vitamin Supplements

- *Fat soluble vitamins;* Such as Vitamin A,D,E and K
- *Water soluble vitamins :* Such as B-complex group and Vitamin C

2. Mineral Supplements

- Macro minerals: Such as Calcium, Phosphorus, magnesium, sodium, potassium and sulphur
- Micro minerals: Such as manganese, zinc, iron, copper and iodine.
- Trace elements: Such as selenium, cobalt, molybdenum and chromium.
- Essential amino acids: Such as Lysine, Methionine and trptophan
- Protein hydrolysates: A pre-digested protein, such as hydrolysed feather meal, hair, etc.
- Liver extract: Supplies essential nutrients in the most assilamiable form.
- Liver yeast and yeast extract: Supplies essential nutrients such as enzymes and unidentified growth factors.
- Fermentable by-products: Supply various essential nutrients, and UGF.

b) Non-nutrient Feed Additives

This group of feed additives do not have any direct nutritional role, but are added to the feed in order to reduce the mortality and morbidity due to various diseases and stress factors, improve the feed efficiency by better digestion, absorption and utilization of nutrients; enhance the colour, flavour, consistency and quality of feed and improve the shelf life of the feed by preventing caking, moulds, mustiness, oxidation and other physical, chemical and microbiological degradation.

Classification and Uses of Non-nutritive Feed Additive

Based on their nature and functions the non-nutritive feed additive may be classified as follows:

- Antibiotic: They are used to control sub-clinical bacterial infections and thereby boost the performance. Ex. Tetracycline, lincomycin, bacitricin, flavomycin, avilamycin, zinc bactricin, virginomycin, etc.
- Non-antibiotic microbial supplement: They check bacterial infections and promote the performance. Ex. Furazolidione, chlorhydroxyquioline.
- Mould inhibitors: They prevent mould growth and production of toxins. Ex. Gentian violet, copper sulphate, propionic acid, calcium propionate
- Coccidiostats: They prevent the outbreak of coccidiosis .Ex. Dinitro-ortho-toluamide, salinomycin, ionophores.
- Anti-parasitic additives: They check various parasitic infections.Ex. Dichlorophan, Niclosamide, etc.
- Anti-oxidants: These are used to prevent oxidative rancidity of fats present in feed ingredients. Ex. BHT, BHA, Ethoxyquin, Vitamin E, Selinium.
- Enzymes: These are added to feed in order to help in digestion. Ex. Protease, lipase, cellulose, amylase, etc.
- Arsenicals: Arsenicals (0.01% or less) promote the growth rate.
- Absorbents: They absorb toxins and prevent their absorption from the intestines. Ex. Bentonite, sodium alginate, lignin.
- Pellet binders: These are used for pelleting the feed in preparation of crumbled feed. Ex. Bentonite, sodium alginate, lignin sulphate.
- Emulsifiers: They increase the surface area of fat for digestion and absorption. Ex. Lecithin.

- Deodorant agents: They reduce the ammonia production in the litter. Ex. Yucca extracts.
- Aromatic/ Flavouring agents: They are added to improve the flavour.
- Pigments: They impart attractive colour to the feed as well as to the products, such as Yolk and skin. Ex. Canthaxanthin, Leutin, Zeaxanthin
- Herbal preparations: They tone up the liver, protect against nephro-toxicity, and stimulate immune system. Ex. Extracts of herbs
- Performance boosters: They improve the overall performance of the birds. Ex.Nitrovin, avoprin
- Immuno stimulants: They stimulate the antibody production, cell mediated immunity.Ex. Tetrahydropheny, levomisole.

Anti-nutritional Factors and Toxins

Anti-nutritional factors or anti-nutrients are the substances found in the feed ingredients that have the potential to adversely affect health, growth and productive performance of the bird. These may include compounds of both plant (endogenous) and microbial origin (exogenous). The plant origin may affect the digestion, absorption and metabolism of nutrients, some important are given in Table 5. However, these anti-nutrients may be removed, though partially, by using various methods like heat treatment, soaking in water, ammunition, solvent extraction, etc.

Table 4: Some anti-nutrients of plant origin

S.No	Anti-nutrients	Occurrence
1.	Tryprin inhibitors Antigenic proteins Protease inhibitors	Soyabean
2.	Haemagglutinins (Lectins)	Legume seeds (Castor bean, kidney bean, Soyabean)
3.	Cyanogens	Cassava root
4.	Glucosinolates	Rapseed
5.	Gossypol	Cotton seed
6.	Phyto-oestrogens	Clover, Lucernes, Soyabean

Mycotoxins

Mycotoxins are those secondary metabolites of fungi that have the capacity to impair poultry health, productivity or sometimes death. No region escapes this silent killer. According to the FAO, approximately 25% of worlds grain supply is contaminated by mycotoxins. Common myctoxins occurring in feeds are given in Table 3. Contamination may occur during harvesting processing and storage of feed stuffs or whenever environmental conditions are appropriate for the spoilage fungi. Moisture content and ambient temperature may be key determinants of fungal colonization and mycotoxin production.

Table 5: Common mycotoxins occurring in poultry feeds

Mycotoxins	**Fungal Species**
Aflatoxins	Aspergillus flavus, A. Parasiticus
Ochratoxin A	A.Ochraceus, Pencillium viridicatum P. Cyclopium
Zearakone	F. Culmorum; F. Graminearum
T-2 toxin	F. Sportrichiodes; F. prae
Fumonisma, moniformin, fusariac acid	
Diacetoxyscirpenol	F. moniliforme F. sporotrichiodes; F. Graminearum
Deoxynivalenol	A. Flavus
Cyclopiazonic acid	P. citrinum; P expansum
Citrinin	P. citrinum, P expansum
Patulin	P. expansum
Citreviridin	P. Citreo-viride

Feed formulation required following information:

1. Composition of feed ingredients commonly used
2. Nature or type of feed
3. Cost and availability of feed ingredients
4. Ingredient inclusion levels and anti-nutritional factors.
5. Acceptability and physical conditions of ingredients
6. Nutrient requirement of poultry
7. Average daily feed consumption of birds
8. Interaction of nutrients
9. Environmental temperature
10. Cost of final products i.e. eggs and poultry meal

Following methods can do feed formulation:

A. By hand calculation

It is possible to design simple diet by hand. The fewer nutrients, such as ME, crude protein, calcium, phosphorous, etc. taken into consideration. Limited number of feed stuffs can be used. But it is still long and tedious process to formulate a diet. This is because substituting one feedstuff for another change all the nutrients in a diet. For a commercial diet with more than 15 feedstuffs and ten nutrients to take into consideration, the possible number of combinations becomes almost infinite. If we then wish to make it least cost diet, it becomes quite clear that we need to apply computers for this task.

B. By using Pearson square

If it is desired to achieve a set percentage of a nutrient in final feed using two ingredients only, Pearson square can be used. It is simple, direct and easy method. It permits quick substitution of feed ingredients in keeping price fluctuations, without disturbing protein content. It is a method of balancing protein requirements, with no consideration given to minerals, vitamins and other nutrient requirements. This technique cannot be used for more than one nutrient and certainly cannot be used to formulate least cost rations.

C. Simultaneous equation method

Rations are formulated by using two sources and one nutrient quickly through the solving of simultaneous equation. Two nutrients can be used.

D. The 2x2 matrix method

E. Computerized feed formulations

Trial and error formulation and linear programming are commonly used with computers for formulating the ration.

Table 6: Composition of Feed for broiler and Layer poultry (in% by weight)

Ingredients of feed	Broiler feed(1-6 weeks)	Grower feed(7-20 weeks)	Layer feed
Yellow Maize	25.0	28.0	30.0
Rice polish	26.0	26.0	20.0
Barley or Oat	7.0	7.0	10.0
Wheat bran	7.0	7.0	8.0
Groundnut cake	18.0	16.0	15.0
Maize gluten powder	5.0	5.0	5.0
Fish meal	6.0	5.0	4.0
Meat meal	3.0	3.0	4.0
Bone meal	1.0	1.0	1.0
Calcium	1.5	1.5	2.5
Salt	0.5	0.5	0.5

Maximum Level of Inclusion of Feed Ingredients

Each ingredient has its maximum level of inclusion in the diet. Inclusion of an ingredient beyond the maximum level may induce imbalance of nutrients, difficulty in feed formulation and may reduce the performance of the birds due to presence of anti nutritional factor beyond tolerance level. Cost is also one of the factors imposing an upper limit on the inclusion of feed ingredients.

Table 7: Maximum levels of inclusion of feed inclusions in poultry diets

Ingredients	Level of inclusions %	
	Chicks	Growers / Layers
Energy Sources		
Maize	60	60
Wheat	50	50
Barley	20	40
Bajra	50	50
Oat	10	20
Sorghum (White)	25	40
Molasses	5	10
Rice polish	40	40
Rice polish (deoiled)	20	20
Rice bran	10	20
Wheat bran	10	15
Tapioca meal	25	25
Hominy feed	10	10
Poultry manure meal	10	10
Protein Sources		
Groundnut cake	40	40
Groundnut cake (deoiled)	20	20
Soyabean meal	40	40
Sesame cake	20	20
Safflower cake	20	20
Linseed meal	20	30

Cottonseed meal	5	5
Mustard cake	10	10
Maize gluten feed	20	20
Maize gluten meal	20	20
Fish meal	15	10
Meat meal	5	10
Bone meal	5	5
Liver meal	10	10
Feather meal	5	5
Poultry by-product meal	5	5
Hatchery by-product meal	5	5
Meat cum bone meal	6	6
Skim milk dried	3	3

Different Types of Poultry Feeds

Poultry feeds are of following six types:

1. Broiler Pre-starter

A ration to be fed to commercial broiler chicks up to the age of 0-10 days.

2. Broiler starter

A ration to be fed to commercial broiler chicks up to the age of 11-25 days.

3. Broiler finisher

A ration to be fed to commercial broiler chicks from 26 days till marketing.

4. Chick feed

A ration to be fed to chicks up to the age of 8 weeks.

5. Grower feed

A ration to be fed to growing chicks from 9-20 weeks.

6. Layer feed

A ration to be fed to laying birds from 20 weeks onwards.

7. Breeder feed

A ration to be fed to laying birds maintained for the production of hatching eggs.

System of Poultry Feeding

A well balanced ration improperly fed will not give the most satisfactory results unless proper method is used. Some of the popular methods of feeding poultry are given below:

Free choice system of feeding

This system had been in vague during the older days of poultry keeping. By this method, the birds are allowed to have their required individual ingredient kept before them in separate hoppers. This system permits birds to consume ingredient, as they wish to balance the ration according to individual needs.

Mash and grain feeding system

This system involves feeding of grain or grain mixture along with balanced mash and is regarded as a slightly better method than the previous. By this one can increase or decrease the protein level as desired. Unless by this method, the layers get a mixture of cereal grains as the scratch portion of their diet and a mash made up of ground grains to which protein, mineral and vitamin supplements are added.

Complete mash feeding system (All mash method)

Now-a-days it is the choice set method of feeding poultry. The mash is fed either dry or wet. Here, the texture of dry mash is important and all the ingredients are ground to appropriate particle size mixed in required proportion and fed as a single balanced mixture. This method is desirable for all types of poultry grown under litter and cage system. By this, the birds can not have the opportunity to have selective eating. In the wet mash system, the dry mash is well-dampened and wetted with water. This practice involves extra labour. On the other hand, wet mash feeding is reported to improve feed consumption during the hotter months of the year and it reduces feed wastage. It may be impracticable to adopt this system, where large flocks to be fed.

Pellet feeding

In this method, regular complete mash is first prepared and then rolled into small cylindrical masses called pellets, in a pelleting mill. It is very widely used in western countries. It allows less wastage of feed and does not permit the birds to pick some of the ingredients of their choice and leave others. Lack of dustiness is another advantage of pellet feeding. Improvement in growth rate and feed utilization has also been claimed by some workers. The main drawback of this system is that pellets are expensive. In some cases, cannibalism is also a problem with pellet feeding.

Controlled or restricted feeding

Several types of feed restriction programme can be followed. It is usually followed from 8-20 weeks of age, i.e., during the growing period. Sometimes sexual maturity of growing pullet is retarded in order to produce larger eggs even during the initial phase of the production or to be obtain more eggs during as particular season. The effects of feed restriction of growers may be summarized as follows:

1. Growers fed restrict diets end up with a lower total feed consumption for the rearing and laying phases combined and thus, feed costs are relatively reduced.
2. Total feed conversion efficiency for egg production are superior in restricted feed flocks than in bird full fed during the grower phase.
3. Restricted feeding results in higher mortality of chickens during the rearing phase, those these losses are balanced by a decreased mortality in the laying period.
4. Growers fed restricted diets have high peak of egg production as compared to those fed ad libitum during the grower phase.

Formulation of Economic and Efficient Ration

Following information is necessary for the formulation of rations:

1. Requirements of nutrients in the diet to be formulated
2. Feed composition tables
3. Maximum level of inclusion of feed ingredients

Nutrient requirement for the poultry bird

The requirement for a given nutrient is the minimum quantity of that nutrient, when all other nutrients are supplied in adequate quantities that will maintain normal growth and reproduction and at the same time prevent the development of symptoms of nutritional deficiency. The accurate way to express the nutrient requirement is in amount per day per animal. Poultry are fed in a group. It is, therefore, not practicable to express the requirement in amounts per day per animal. The bureau of Indian standards has laid down standard specification for starting, growing and laying chicken feed to serve as a guide for the feed manufacturers and poultry keepers. There is no single feed formula which can be claimed to be best in all cases, but the feed should fulfill the nutritional requirements adequately consistent with economy. The dietary allowances of a given nutrient are the quantity of the nutrient that is given to the bird. A reasonable allowance makes no provision for a margin of safety. In most cases, allowances will exceed the requirements for several reasons.

- To provide a margin of safety
- To allow for stability problem. Some nutrients are not stable; for example several of fat soluble vitamins are subject to oxidative destruction.
- To allow for variations in composition of feed ingredients. These vary due to climatic conditions.
- To avoid loss during storage.
- To allow for increased concentration of the ration especially, if added fat is used in the formula.

Feed formulation

In current situations, computers are utilized extensively to formulate least cost poultry ration using linear programming but where such facilities are not available, we have to compute the formula by looking into the common poultry feed ingredients available in the locally and their cost. There is no single formula which can be considered best for rapid and efficient growth and egg production. Quality and cost of feed ingredients will greatly affect the formula of economic rations. The objective should be minimum cost. The essential considerations in the formulation of poultry rations are nutritive adequacy and economy. Feed should contain proper proportion of protein, carbohydrates, fats, minerals and vitamins. The best result should be obtained with lowest possible cost.

- Cereals form the principal ingredient of poultry ration feeding a mixture of cereals or their by-products instead of any single one is advisable since this may help in making up the deficiency of others and also help in reducing the cost of feed.
- A combination of both animal and vegetable protein should be included to supply adequate balance of amino acids while keeping the cost low.
- Minerals and vitamins should be supplemented in required proportions.
- The feed should contain the necessary bulk to satisfy hunger. Although fibre is poorly utilized a certain amount of it is required in the ration (6-8%).
- During selection of ingredients the digestibility and palatability are of great importance since feed utilization depends upon their factors.

Methods of Evaluating Poultry Feedstuffs

1. Appearance

It gives an indication of its feeding value. Products that's off colour or brown instead of their normal colour indicate poor quality of the product. Caked or lumpy material may indicate mouldy or wet product.

2. Odour

This may also help in judging its quality. For example, sore smell of molasses indicates the possibilities of toxic nature of the product. Rancid meat meal or fish meal will have a strong pungent odour.

3. Microscopic analysis

Here, one may examine the feedstuff spread out in a thin layer on a white sheet of a paper with the aid of a hand lens. One can detect by this method the amount of fibre or bulk in feedstuff. This method with the help of odour and appearance will give fair guidance in detecting the quality of feed ingredient.

4. Chemical analysis

This includes the determination of proximate principles, such as ash, moisture, crude protein, crude fat and crude fibre. This is a better method than all the previous method. However, it is not a completely reliable method since materials may have a good chemical composition but may be poor in biological value.

5. Feeding trials

This is the best measure of value of a feed stuff or ration. It will determine whether it is palatable or not. Tests may be designed to measure its digestibility which is highly desirable, although time consuming.

Storage of Feed

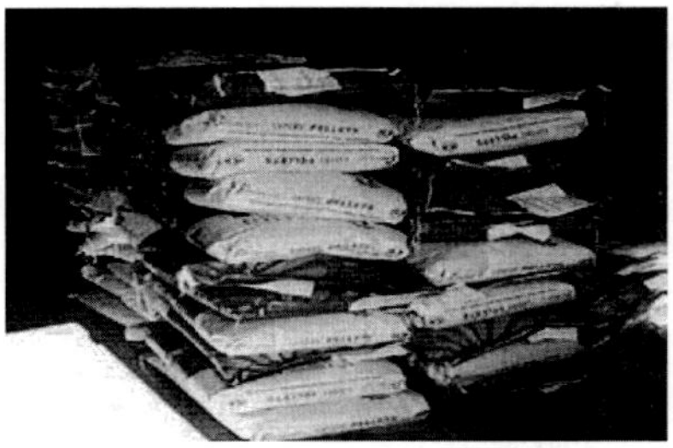

Storage of poultry feed

Storing poultry feeds sounds straight forward enough but there are a number of pitfalls to watch out for, especially for the newcomer. One needs a well-ventilated, cool, dry shed or similar to store it in. To prevent the feed from absorbing moisture, it should not be stored on a cold concrete floor, even if it is a dry floor because it will absorb moisture from condensation. Using a wooden pallet is the preferred method of storing bags of feed but you can improvise using some pieces of wood, if you can't get hold of one. This allows air to circulate underneath them and prevents the condensation problem.

The next problem is vermin. Rats and mice will soon eat their way through your precious supplies, so if you can, ensure rats cannot get into the storage area and if mice can get in, leave traps set nearby and check them regularly. When setting mouse traps, chocolate is particularly effective and lures mice away from the smell of your poultry feeds. Rat runs and holes should be well-baited outside or you should have humane cage traps set and covered over against walls which should keep them away from your feeds. If you want to store 2 or 3 bags, then a good idea is to use a galvanized bins or containers. These are well worth investing in and will prevent rats and mice getting to your food. Rats can chew through wood and plastic but they can't get through galvanized steel.

The cheapest option for a bag or two is a plastic waste bin. This will stop mice (the most common problem), so providing you don't have a lot of rats in the area, you should find this a satisfactory solution. For larger quantities that can't be stored in galvanized bins like the 50 bags placed on a concrete floor. Feed is stored on wooden pallets and a gap is left between the bags and the walls of the shed to allow ventilation.

There are metal grills at high level that allow air movement. The shed must be located in the shade, so it doesn't heat up too much in the sun or the nutrients in the food will be destroyed.

Storage Time

Finally, keep an eye on the best before dates on the bags of feed. Whilst the feed seems to look alright, many of the nutrients and vitamins will have depleted after the best before date and chick crumbs or growers pellets that may contain added drugs may not be as effective.3-6 months is the normal length of time you get, when buying feed, so make sure you can use the amount you buy before the best before date.

Tips on storing feed

The following guidelines will help to ensure that feed remains fresh, palatable and in optimum condition:

- Store feed in a cool, dry place. Heat and sunlight will dry the feed making it less palatable, and heat combined with moisture from the feed will provide ideal conditions for spoilage.
- Feed sacks that are stored on pallets should have enough room so that air can circulate freely around the sacks. Care should also be taken that the feed sacks are not stacked against walls which will also damage the sack and feed inside.
- Opened feed sacks should be resealed between uses or put into lidded bins. If feed bins are used, the bin should always be thoroughly cleaned before it is refilled. Old feed left in the bottom of bins provides the ideal breeding ground for mite.
- The feed room itself should be kept clean and tidy, as spilt feed will encourage vermin.

- If you have several sacks of feed make sure you always check the labels and use the oldest feed first. As feed is a perishable product, it is important to use it as soon as possible after purchase.
- The 'best before' date is an indication of the nutritional integrity of the feed, i.e. the vitamin and nutrient feeding value will be at the declared levels. However, it does not provide a guarantee that the feed will still be fit to feed after a period of time. A poorly stored bag of feed can 'go off' in less than a week, if stored incorrectly.

❑❑❑

Chapter **12**

Poultry Health and Diseases

Maintaining the poultry birds in good shape and health is equally important since it may affect the production and productivity of the birds, which directly affects the economics of the farm. Therefore, due importance should be given to the poultry health care. Generally, diseases are caused by various factors like microbes, parasites, nutrition, management and many other factors. Microbes like bacteria, virus, fungus, etc. cause most of the diseases. These organisms are so small that they are not visible to our eyes. They spread rapidly mostly through contact, air, feed and water. Therefore, in order to run the poultry farm in a profitable way, it is essential to follow many biosecurity measures to prevent the occurrence and spread of these diseases.

Identification of Sick Birds

When a layer or broiler bird gets sick, it will affect its feed and water intake, which in turn affects the growth and productivity (egg and meat). The birds also show different physical and behavioural signs/ symptoms. It is essential to regularly, observe the birds for both physical and behavioural signs for identifying the sick birds. Once the sick birds are identified, they should be removed from the flock to prevent spreading of the disease. The major differences between the healthy and sick birds are tabulated below:

Table 1: Difference between healthy and sick birds

Sl. No.	Parameters	Healthy Birds	Sick or Diseased Birds
1)	Alertness	Active and alert; Highly responsive	Dull and less active; Less responsive
2)	Feed and water intake	Show interest	Show no or less interest
3)	Behaviour	Move freely	Separate away from the flock or huddle together
4)	Coughing or Sneezing or Panting	Absent	Present
5)	Head	Normal and stiff	Bent towards the body

6)	Eyes	Open, Bright and clean with no discharge	Closed, Cloudy or Dull with discharge
7)	Comb and Wallet	Hot, red or pink colour, normal size	Cold, pale or blue or black colour, Swollen
8)	Nostril	Clean, Dry and open	Blocked with discharge
9)	Beak	Normal shape, Stiff, Closed	Twisted or bent, Soft and rubbery, Open
10)	Skin	Shiny and pink	Dull and yellowish or pale
11)	Feathers	Shiny, clean and fluffy, No ticks/lice/fleas	Ruffled and dirty, ticks/lice/fleas may be present
12)	Vent or cloaca	Clean with no abnormal discharge	Dirty (soiled) with mucous or bloody discharge
13)	Toes	Straight	Bent or twisted
14)	Droppings	Semi-solid	Green or bright yellow or bloody with diarrhoea
15)	Gait (Movement)	Stiff and erect	Unable to stand or move properly, Limping
16)	Egg Production	Normal	No or less production
17)	Egg Size and Shape	Normal size and shape	Small size, abnormal shape
18)	Egg Shell	Normal thickness	No shell or thin shell
19)	Body Temperature	40.6 to 43.0°C (105 to 109°F)	Above normal
20)	Heart Rate	250 – 300 beats per minute	Above normal
21)	Respiration Rate	15-40 breaths/counts per minute	Above normal

It is essential to go around the sheds at least twice in a day, observe the birds carefully without disturbing them and identify the sick birds so that they can be removed from the flock to prevent spreading of diseases.

Common Diseases of Poultry

Disease mainly refers to discomfort. If a bird is affected by a disease condition, it feels uneasiness and will not be able to perform its normal functions (e.g. egg production) to its full capacity. The most common causes of disease in poultry are microbes (bacteria, virus, fungi and protozoa), parasites, nutrition deficiency and metabolic disorders. Important diseases of poultry, their causes, mode of transmission and common signs are tabulated below:

Table 2: Important diseases of poultry

Sl. No.	Disease	Birds commonly affected	Mode of transmission	Common signs and symptoms
A) Bacterial Diseases:				
1)	*E. coli* infections	Broilers and layers	Feed, water, litter, hatching eggs	Swelling and infection of the nasal region, watery or yellowish droppings
2)	Infectious Coryza	Broilers and layers	Direct contact, air and contaminated drinking water	Off-feed (show no or less interest in feeding), swelling of face and wattles, nasal discharge, sound while breathing, diarrhoea with bad smell/ odour
3)	Chronic Respiratory Disease (CRD)	Broilers and layers	Contact, air, contaminated equipment, hatching eggs	Decreased feed intake, sound while breathing, discharge from nostril, coughing, sneezing, loss of body weight
4)	Bacillary White Diarrhoea (Pullorum Disease)	Layers, Newly hatched chicks	Hatching eggs; eating of egg and dead birds, wound infection and contaminated feed and water	Weakness, off-feed, huddling together with closed eyes, shrill cry while passing faeces/ droppings (defecating), chalky white diarrhoea in chicks. Depression, off-feed, diarrhoea, dehydration and decreased egg production in adults.
5)	Fowl Cholera	Broilers and layers	Contact with contaminated crates, feed, bags, shoes, and other equipment	Fever, gasping, coughing, sneezing, difficulty in breathing, yellow or green diarrhoea, ruffled feathers, lameness and swelling of joints of leg/ wing/ comb
B) Viral Diseases:				
6)	Avian Influenza (Bird flu)	Broilers and layers	Direct contact, Air, contact with contaminated equipment and farm staff.	Depression, decreased feed intake, swollen blue combs and wattles, coughing, sneezing, diarrhoea, nervous signs, sudden death and mortality (death) may go up to 100%
7)	Infectious Bursal Disease (Gumboro disease)	Broilers and layers	Water, feed and droppings	Off-feed, depression, dehydration, shivering, ruffled feathers, whitish or watery diarrhoea, and pecking of vent/anus
8)	Ranikhet Disease (Newcastle disease)	Broilers and layers	Air, feed and water, Direct or indirect contact	Difficulty in breathing, Sneezing, gasping, nasal discharge, Greenish diarrhoea, twisting of neck, paralysis of legs/wings and sudden death within 4 to 8 days

9)	Egg Drop Syndrome (EDS 76)	Layers	Hatchery	Loss of colour in coloured eggs, thin and soft shelled eggs or shell less eggs, sudden drop in egg production, small eggs and eggs with poor interior quality
10)	Fowl Pox	Layers	Injured or broken skin	Wart like pox lesions/swellings on the head and non-feathered regions like legs, feet, eyelids, comb, wattles and vent, coryza-like signs are also noticed
11)	Marek's Disease	Broilers and Layers	Air, direct or indirect contact	Enlargement of internal organs, paralysis of legs, skin lesions
12)	Infectious Bronchitis (IB)	Layers	Air, direct or indirect contact	Severe reduction in growth, decreased feed consumption, Respiratory discomfort like gasping, coughing, sneezing, tracheal rales and nasal discharge in chicks. Respiratory symptoms, reduced egg production, especially towards the latter part of the egg production, production of soft-shelled, misshapen or rough shelled eggs in adults.
13)	Lymphoid Leucosis	Layers	Direct or indirect contact, through hatching eggs	Off-feed, pale and bluish combs, loss of body condition, enlarged abdomen and internal organs, nervous sign, watery droppings.
C. Fungal Diseases:				
14)	Aflatoxicosis	Broilers and layers	Feed with toxins	Reduced growth and sudden death
15)	Brooder Pneumonia	Layer	Air, Direct or indirect contact	Off-feed, gasping or coughing and rapid loss of body weight
D. Parasitic/Protozoal Disease:				
16)	Coccidiosis	Broilers and layers	Feed and water	Birds become pale, dull, move away from the flock to a corner, sleeping while standing, bloody droppings, ruffled feathers, poor growth, reduced egg production and loss of body condition
E. Management Related Diseases:				
17)	Leg Disorders	Broilers	Various causes	Bending of legs, impaired walking or refusal to walk
18)	Breast Blisters	Broilers and Layers	Poor feathering, hard flooring, increased sitting	Nodule like swelling (blisters) in the breast region
19)	Cage Layer Fatigue	Layer	Rearing in cages	Inability to stand, Thinning of long bones, easy breaking of bones

Deworming and vaccination

Deworming and vaccination are two important precautionary control measures to be followed in a poultry farm in order to maintain the birds in a healthy and disease free condition.

a) Deworming: Parasites particularly the worms also cause huge economic loss to the poultry farmers. These worms once enter the body of the birds through contaminated feed and water will affect the health of the birds and there by resulting in poor growth rate and decreased feed consumption & productivity and sometimes cause mortality (death). Therefore, it is important to prevent the occurrence of worm infestation in birds. Worm infestation can be prevented by deworming the birds regularly. Deworming is the process of administering/ giving an anti-parasitic drugs to the birds in order to eliminate or prevent the worm infestation.

b) Vaccination: For making the poultry farm profitable, it is advisable to follow a famous saying "Prevention is better than cure". It is always economical to prevent the occurrence of disease rather than treating the diseased birds. Disease can be prevented by many ways. The most important and economical ways of preventing some of the deadly diseases like Raniket's disease or Gumboro disease is by administering vaccines. Vaccines are preparations, when administered/ given to the birds at an appropriate time and dose (quantity) will help in preventing the occurrence of that particular disease. Vaccines act by stimulating the bird's body immune system. Therefore, even if the vaccine bird is exposed to the disease causing organisms, the immune system developed due to vaccine will help the bird to protect itself from the disease.

Vaccination in Broilers

Broilers are reared only for about 35 to 42 days of age and vaccinated against the diseases prevalent in area of poultry farm. Generally, broilers are vaccinated against only 2-3 important diseases as tabulated below:

Table 3: Vaccination Schedule in Broiler Chicken

Name of disease	Age at 1st vaccination	Doses of vaccine	Route of vaccination
Marek's disease	1st day	0.2 ml (Using sterile ½ inch needle of 20-22 gauge)	Done at Hatchery. Nasal or Subcutaneous route in the lower neck region
Newcastle or Ranikhet Disease (F1 strain)	5-7th day	1-2 drop	Ocular or Nasal
Infectious Bursal Disease/Gumboro	14-16th day	1-2 drop	Drinking water
Raniket (Lasota)	28-30th day	1-2 drop	Drinking water

Vaccination in Layers

The layers are reared till they are of 72 weeks of age. Therefore, they require vaccination against many vaccines and in repeated doses as tabulated below:

Table 4: Vaccination Schedule in layer chicken

Age of the bird	Disease	Route
1st day	Marek's disease	Used as Hatchery Vaccination. Nasal or Subcutaneous route in the lower neck region
5th- 7th day	Raniket Disease	Ocular or Nasal
10th day	Infectious Bronchitis	Water
14th day	Infectious Bursal Disease	Ocular or nasal
24th day	Infectious Bursal Disease	Drinking water
28th- 30th day	Ranikhet Disease + Infectious Bronchitis	Ocular or nasal or Drinking water
5th- 6th week	Coryza*	Sub-cutaneous injection (Neck)
7th week	Fowl pox	Sub-cutaneous injection (wing stab)
9th- 10th week	Ranikhet Disease	Sub-cutaneous injection (wing web)
12th week	Infectious Bronchitis	Ocular or nasal or Drinking water
13th- 14th week	Infectious Coryza*	Sub-cutaneous injection (Neck)
17th week	Ranikhet Disease	Sub-cutaneous injection (Neck)
Layer House	Ranikhet Disease	Every 3 months - drinking water
* Not compulsory (Optional) Ocular: A drop into the eye Nasal: A drop into the nostril S/c: Below the skin		

Precautions to be followed before, during and after vaccination

- Vaccine should be purchased only from a reliable source.

- Batch numbers, date of manufacture/expiry date and supplier's details should be recorded properly for future reference.
- Expired vaccines should neither be purchased nor used.
- Store the vaccine at the temperature of 2-8°C; they should neither be frozen nor kept above 8°C.
- Vaccine should not be exposed directly to sunshine or extreme weather conditions.
- Vaccination should be carried out during cooler part of the day.
- All healthy birds should be vaccinated. Sick birds should not be vaccinated.
- While administering water-based vaccines, water should be withdrawn for 2-3 hours before administering the vaccine.
- Adequate drinker space should be provided.
- Vaccine should be administered as per the instructions/ recommendations of the manufacturer.
- When a vaccine vial is opened, complete contents should be used at once. The vaccine should be opened and mixed just before administering the vaccine.
- The vaccinating equipment must be sterilized. Chemical disinfectants should not be used for sterilization, as it will affect the effectiveness of the vaccine.
- Premixed vaccine should be carried in a flask filled with ice water and should be used as quickly as possible; preferably, within two to three hours.
- Empty vials, left-over vaccines and other material containing the vaccine must be burnt and destroyed properly.

Administration of Medicines / Drugs

Medicines/drugs for the treatment and control of diseases can be given to birds in different ways. The method of administration of medicine/drug/vaccine depends on the type and severity of the disease, age or condition of the birds, type of drug/vaccine, etc. The different techniques employed for administering medicine to chicken are described below:

a) Oral: In this method, medicines are given to birds through mouth. It includes administration of drugs/medicines in feed and water. Only few drugs/medicines like mineral/vitamin supplements, growth promoters, antibiotics for preventing the occurrence of disease, etc. are given by this method.

b) Nasal: Here, medicines are given to birds through nostril in the form of droplets or spray using a dropper. Few vaccines are administered by this method.

c) Ocular: In this method, medicines are given to birds into the eyes in the form of eye drops using a dropper. Some of the vaccines are administered through this method.

b) Injection: Medicines/drugs/vaccines are administered directly into the body of the birds either into the muscles (intramuscular), under the skin (subcutaneous) or in the webbing of the wing (wing web) in this method. Administration of medicines through injection method should be done only by a qualified veterinary practitioner. Always check for the manufacturer's instruction in the medicine/vaccine vial especially regarding the mode of injection.

- Intra-muscular: In intra-muscular injection, the medicine/ vaccine is injected into the muscles located in the neck or thigh region.
- Subcutaneous: In this method, medicine/vaccine is deposited in the layer between skin and muscle. Mostly vaccines are administered by this method.
- Wingweb: Here, medicine/vaccineis deposited in the webbing of the wing. Few vaccines are administeredby this method.

Note

- Do not treat the birds yourself. It is always advisable to follow the instructions of the registered veterinary practitioner with respect to the administration of drugs/medicines and vaccines.
- It is important to note that the method of administration of drugs/ medicines and vaccines should be strictly followed as per the method and instructions suggested by the manufacturer of the medicine or registered veterinarian.
- Changes in the method of administration of drugs/vaccines will not yield the desirable effects/results and may sometimes even cause serious consequences or even lead to death of the bird(s).

❒❒❒

Chapter **13**

Disease Investigation

Disease investigation requires knowledge of what to expect at what age and how to detect what is abnormal for the flock. It is important to be familiar with the normal production parameters or standards for the breed. When health problems are seen or suspected in a flock, veterinary advice should be sought immediately.

A systematic approach is required when troubleshooting health issues are in the farm. The following are the things to look at:

- Feed : Availability, consumption, distribution, palatability, nutritional content, contaminants and toxins.
- Light : adequate for growth and development, uniform exposure and intensity.
- Litter : Material used depth, distribution, moisture level, pathogen load, toxins and contaminant.
- Air : Speed, availability, humidity, temperature, contaminants (ammonia level and toxins) and barriers.
- Water : Availability, consumption, distribution, source, contaminants and toxins, pathogen load, additives and sanitizers.
- Space : Bird density, limiting obstacles, limiting equipment, feed and water availability.
- Sanitation : Hygiene of premises, pest control, maintenance, cleaning and disinfection practices.
- Security : Biosecurity risks.

After becoming familiar with various diseases and ailments of poultry, the next step is to get their diagnosis as soon as possible. This is because the course of action will depend on the nature of the disease. One should not delay the diagnosis for any reason, when a disease threatens, otherwise it may get out of hand before diagnosis is made.

Therefore, getting a diagnosis as quickly as possible is of the greatest importance. It is not possible to treat a disease or check its harmful effects, but to plan effectively for future, it is important to identify all diseases that occur.

A multi-pronged approach is made in this chapter to arrive at a diagnosis. A key to good disease diagnosis is to diagnose the most important flock problem, rather than getting too much occupied with individual bird disorders. The best approach is to begin with history. Get a complete history the disease and all related events leading to the outbreak. The more information is collected, the more easily one can proceed at solving the problem.

A. How to carry out a field investigation

While carrying out a field investigation, one must always remember that common things occur commonly. Therefore, one should concentrate on probabilities than possibilities. The following basic points must be borne in mind:

- The problem lies at the farm rather than in the laboratory.
- The diagnosis should indicate the major production problems, rather than just an obvious cause of mortality.
- The preliminary diagnosis may require only good observation and scissors. Laboratory confirmation may follow.
- Without adequate records, a reliable diagnosis may not be possible.
- Record and report accurately and fairly.

Basically there are two categories of problems that require investigation:

1. The postmortem-based, laboratory-confirmed, relatively easy and straight forward problems for making diagnosis of some disease conditions and possibly prescribing specific treatment.
2. The in-depth (very thorough) investigation to find out the underlying cause of an infectious disease, or to attempt to define a more vague, possibly a multi-factorial condition and determine its origin and treatment.

History

The first step in any investigation is to obtain and record a detailed history. This needs time. While carrying out an on-farm or on-site investigation, the following guidelines may be observed:

- Collect all the history and write it down. Records of mortality, egg production, hatchability, etc. may be taken.
- Walk around the site or farm and observe. Get to know the people involved, evaluate them and gain their confidence.
- A drop in egg production may be caused by theft of eggs and increased feed consumption or by theft of feed.
- Important questions should be put on more than one occasion, but in different ways and to different staff during the course of investigation in order to get overall idea.
- It is essential to know the normal before abnormal can be appreciated.
- Postmortem examination forms only one part of any such investigation.

Problems

Usually, the problems are of two types:

1. Mortality (deaths) morbidity (sickness) in chicks, growers or adult birds.
2. Drop in production and/or quality of either growth (body weight, feed conversion ratio), or eggs.

Investigation of disease involving mortality and morbidity

The case history, a postmortem examination, and usually laboratory investigation are required. A visit to the farm/site may be helpful.

History

The following information should be collected for routine investigation of any disease outbreak:

- Origin of flock
- Type of bird

- Strain of bird
- System of rearing
- System of management(all-in, all-out, or multi-age)
- Age
- Percentage of sick
- Number of birds in the farm
- Mortality record for the last seven days
- Symptoms of disease.
- Postmortem findings
- Laboratory findings
- Tentative diagnosis
- Immediate recommendations
- Final Diagnosis
- Final treatment.

However, in case of a severe problem, more detailed investigation is necessary. In this regard, the following aspects may be considered:

1. Building and Management

- Size and type of building
- Management system
- Stock density
- Type and condition of litter

2. Equipment

- Brooders, heaters
- Cage design, stocking
- Feeders, drinkers
- Space per bird

3. Ventilation

- Fans: number :type ,condition
- Temperature, air flow, spread of birds on the floor

- Control system in use.
- Variation of temperature

4. Lighting

- Pattern
- Intensity

5. Nutrition

- Type of ration
- Raw materials
- Minerals
- Premix/supplement
- Feed and water system
- Recent change of feed/system/method
- Pellet quality
- Feed and water consumption record

6. Production Details

- Broiler:(weight and feed conversion ratio)
- Layer: Weeks in lay, production percentage/bird/day

7. Disease

- Vaccination details and record
- Previous history of illness in the flock
- Drug treatment record
- Mortality and morbidity record
- Presence of external parasites, worms

Systems of present problem and causes

- External : Feathering, extent/quality, skin/eye/lesions, parasites
- Respiratory : Coughing, sneezing, head shaking, swollen eyes, nasal discharge

- Nervous : Trembling, ataxia, falling, lying down, paralysis, circling, blindness
- Locomotion : Crooked toes, enlarged hocks or other joints, slipped tendon, spread out legs, paralysis, leg trembling, leg weakness
- Digestive : Off-feed, droppings (intestinal: consistency, bloody, white and green
- Body weight : Average, low, normal

Postmortem Examination

Postmortem examination of poultry is essential to determine the cause of death. That is to arrive at a correct diagnosis so that disease outbreak, if any, can be effectively controlled. Postmortem examination should be carried out as early as possible because once putrefiction sets in, then it becomes difficult to identify the tissue changes and isolate the organisms responsible for the disease.

Selection of Birds: Selection of birds is very important. This is because a wrong conclusion of a situation may be arrived at from postmortem carried out on improperly selected birds.

Killing of Birds: Several methods may be used to kill the birds. The following methods may be adopted:

1. Cervical Dislocation.
2. Inhalation Euthanasia.
3. Injection Euthanasia.

Postmortem Technique

When birds are submitted for postmortem examination, they should be placed on its back and examined for any physical deformity, external parasites, discharges from nostrils and eyes, paleness of comb and wattles, dehydration and emaciation. The skin from vent to beak should be cut to expose the internal organs. Lungs, air sacs, etc. should be examined for any abnormalities .Samples should be collected from those organs which show any abnormality. The collected samples may be subjected to following laboratory examination:

- Impression Smear
- Bacterial Culture
- Histopathological Examination

Materials to be Sent to the Laboratory for Disease Diagnosis

A. Viral Diseases

Ranikhet Disease

- Serum samples for serological tests.
- Proventriculus, Intestines, trachea.

Gumboro Disease (Infectious Bursal Disease)

- Bursa and spleen.
- Macerated bursa and serum samples
- Bursa and kidneys in 10% formaline.

Infectious Bronchitis

- Trachea, lungs, air sacs, caecal contents, tonsils, kidneys and oviduct in 50% glycerine.
- Serum samples

Infectious Laryngotrachitis

- Tracheal exudates
- Trachea in 10% formaline
- Serum samples

Fowl Pox

- Pieces from skin and other tissue lesions in 10% formaline
- Smears prepared from the lesions for detection of inclusion bodies.
- Lesions of fowl pox in 50% glycerine.
- Serum samples

Marek's Disease

- Sciatic and brachial nerve
- Liver, spleen, ovary, lungs, proventriculus in 10% formaline
- Feather tip in 50% glycerine saline
- Serum samples

Lymphoid Leukosis

- Pieces of liver, spleen,bursa, thymus, bone marrow, gonads and bracial nerve in 10% formaline
- Impression smears of fresh tumors
- Serum or plasma samples

Avian Influenza

- Liver in 50% glycerine saline
- Pieces of liver in 10% formaline
- Serum samples for serological tests

Leechi Disease

- Pieces of liver in 10% formaline
- Pieces of liver in 50% glycerine

Chicken Infectious Anemia

- Serum samples for serological tests
- Liver Impression smears for detection of antibodies.

B. Bacterial Diseases

Colibacillosis

- Heart, liver and lungs
- Serum samples for serological tests

Infectious Coryza

- Swabs from infraorbital sinus, trachea, and air sacs.
- Serum samples for serological tests

Salmonellosis

- Liver, gall bladder, or yolk sac
- Serum samples for serological tests

Fowl Cholera

- Impression smears from liver and lungs or smears of heart blood.
- Liver, bone marrow, heart blood.

Fowl Typhoid

- Liver, bone marrow, heart blood
- Whole blood and serum for serological tests.

Pullorum Disease

- Liver, spleen and caeca
- Whole blood and serum

Necrotic Enteritis

- Intestinal contents, scrapings of intestinal wall or haemorrhagic lesions

Ulcerative Enteritis: bone marrow, heart blood

- Liver or spleen

Gangrenous Dermatitis

- Exudates of skin and subcutaneous tissue or underlying muscles.

Mycoplasmosis

- Swabs from nasal cavity, air sacs, trachea and lungs as well as exudates aspirated from the infraorbital sinus and joints
- Serum samples for serological tests

C. Fungal Disease

Aspergillosis (Brooder pneumonia)

- Smear from lesions.
- Lesions in the lungs or air sacs.

Mycotoxicosis

Samples (500g) of suspected feed, feed ingredients and mouldy clamps.

Table 1: Disease diagnosis on the basis of symptoms.

Diseases	Symptoms
Marek's Disease	Paralysis of legs and wings
Avian Influenza	Sudden death, bluish discolouration of wattless, comb and shanks
Ascites	Swollen abdomen and congestion of abdominal skin
Coccidiosis	Blood in droppings
Infectious coryza	Nasal discharge, facial oedema, conjunctivitis
Cage layer fatigue	Paralysis of laying birds in cages
Infectious stunting syndrome	Stunting and retarded development
Lysine deficiency	Stunting and retarded development
Riboflavin deficiency	Curled toe paralysis
Swollen head syndrome	Swelling of head, puffy appearance of face and swollen eyes
Thiamine deficiency	Typical star gazing
Egg drop syndrome	Thin shelled, soft shelled, shell less eggs
Infectious Bronchitis	Thin shelled, rough and deformed eggs
Sudden death syndrome	Healthy, fast growing broiler dying on their back with short wing beating
Choline deficiency	Stunting, poor feathering and short, thick bowed legs
Ranikhet Disease	Facial oedema with haemorrhagic conjunctivitis
Infectious Laryngotracheitis	Difficulty in breathing with dried blood around nostrils
Rickets	Stiff-legged gait and progressive lameness

Ranikhet Disease	Pin point haemorrhages on the tips of glands in proventriculus; Haemorrhagic caecal tonsils; white spots of dead tissue on the spleen
Gumboro Disease	Enlarged and swollen bursa, presence of cheesy within the lumen, haemorrahges on the surface of bursa and thighs
Infectious Bronchitis	Caseous plug in the lower trachea or bronchi and air sacs. Lungs are congested and presence of urates in kidneys
Infectious Laryngotrachitis	Trachea is inflamed red and may contain blood.
Fowl Pox	**Skin form** : Pox lesions on comb and wattles. **Diptheric form** : Small white nodules in larynx and trachea
Avian influenza	Marked bluish discolouration of comb and wattles. Severe head swelling and eye discharges, small haemorrhages on the heart and muscles
Mareks Disease	Classical form: Marked enlargement of one or more nerves, mainly sciatic and brachial nerves.
Chicken Infectious Anaemia	Reduction in the size of Thymus and bursa
Inclusion Body Hepatitis	Liver pale, friable and swollen. Small a nd large haemorrhages in the liver and skeletal muscles.
Leechi Disease	Presence of clear fluid in the pericardial sac.
Collibacillosis	Heart, liver and air sacs covered by a layer of white inflammatory
Infectious Coryza	Swelling of the face, Presence of pus or mucus with fibrin in nasal passages and infraorbital sinuses.

Necrotic Enteritis	Small intestine is greatly thickened and shows loose to tightly attached yellow or green layer.
Gangrenous Dermatitis	Affected area is very dark and moist. The tissue is dead and tends to slough.
Ulcerative Enteritis	Severe haemorrhagic enteritis, Ulceration in caeca
Pullorum Disease	**Chicks**: Unabsorbed yolk, Lungs is congested and liver is dark. Foci of dead tissue found in the liver, lungs and heart. **Adult:** Ova is irregular, cystic, deformed, discolouration.
Salmonellosis	Lungs, liver, spleen and kidneys are swollen and congested. Unabsorbed yolk. White areas of dead tissues in the lungs, liver and heart.
Mycoplasmosis	Cheese like inflammatory material in air sacs and lungs
Aspergillosis	Nodules in the nasal passage, trachea and air sacs.
Aflatoxicosis	Enlargement of liver, kidney and spleen. Liver is enlarged yellow and friable with small haemorrhages
Coccidiosis	Caeca is greatly enlarged. And distended with clotted blood.
Gout	**Visceral gout**: Kidney, heart, proventriculus and lungs show urate deposition **Articular gout**: Urate deposition in joints.
Ascites	Presence of a large amount of fluid in abdominal cavity
Fatty liver and kidney syndrome	Liver and kidneys are enlarged, pale and fatty
Fatty liver and Haemorrhagic syndrome	Pools of blood in the abdomen, Liver is enlarged and fatty, friable and light greyish brown to yellow in colour.

❑❑❑

Chapter **14**

Disinfection

A disinfectant is a chemical that destroys disease-producing organisms on contact. To disinfectant is to free from disease-producing organisms (bacteria, viruses, fungi, etc.), or to make them inactive; and disinfection is the act of destroying infectious agents. (To sanitise is to reduce the number of bacteria present and also to prevent them from multiplying).

Disinfectants and disinfection procedures have been widely used for many years in the poultry industry. Natural disinfection agents, such as sunlight, heat, or just simply resting poultry houses, are considered to be of limited use. Increasing evidence of the prolonged survival time of a number of important chicken pathogens (disease-producing organisms) outside the body of the birds, together with an ever-increasing economic pressure for quicker re-stocking of units, has led to a greater dependence on chemical disinfectants.

Properties of a Disinfectant

The lethal action (i.e. causing death) of a disinfectant depends on the chemical composition of the disinfectant and the type of organism. An ideal disinfectant should have all, or most of the following properties:

1. It must be cost-effective and produce benefit to the farmer in terms of improved production. That is, reduced mortality, increased live weight gain, and feed conversion.
2. It must be effective against all the infectious agents (viruses, bacteria, fungi). That is, must have a broad-spectrum actively. It must be effective under farm conditions, organic soiling, hard water and low temperature.
3. It must be safe for humans and animals.
4. It must be soluble in water.

5. It must be readily available.
6. It must be safe to the environment
7. It must be corrode the utensils, fabrics, equipment or fittings.
8. It must be stable, when exposed to air.
9. It should be free from any objectionable or lingering odour.
10. There should be no residual toxicity.
11. There should be no harmful accumulation of any portion of the disinfectant in meat or eggs.

No disinfectant works immediately. All require a certain amount of contact time to be effective. Use of disinfectants at the recommended concentration is important for their effectiveness. All disinfectants are less effective in the presence of organic matter, e.g., faeces, soil, etc. Organic matter interferes with the action of disinfectants by coating the disease-producing organisms and preventing their contact with the disinfectant.

Therefore, for any disinfectant to be effective, it must be applied to surfaces that have been first freed from debris and organic matter by thorough scraping, scrubbing, brushing, and dusting, and washing with soap or detergent solutions. Many disinfectants are highly efficient, but only when first these basic cleaning requirements have been met.

Types of disinfectants

1. Sunlight : It is often a valuable disinfectant, if surface are exposed directly for a sufficient duration. It loses its power to kill germs after it passes through thin film of water dust or ordinary glass. The disinfecting action of it is due to ultraviolet rays.
2. Heat
   i) Hot air : It is an effective means of disinfection but often an expensive one, hence is limited to labortaries.
   ii) Hot water : Almost all utensils of used in poultry can be disinfected by immersion in boiling water for a little more than 5 minutes. It is not satisfactory way for disinfecting floors, as it loses its heat soon.

iii) Steam : It is satisfactory means of disinfection but being expensive, its use as disinfectant is chiefly limited to utensils. It is used under 15 lbs pressure.

iv) Fire : It adds to the total destruction of bacteria and spores, therefore a best means of disposing infecting carcass and litter.

3. Chemicals as disinfectants kill germs by:

    i) Hydrolytic action on cell - e.g. acids, alkalies

    ii) Oxidation action on protoplasm of cell - Potassium permanganate, Hydrogen peroxide

    iii) Protein Coagulation in protoplasm of cell - Alcohol formaldehyde

    iv) Disruption of cell wall and cell membrane - Phenol, cresols polymixin

Various Classes of Disinfectants

There are a variety of disinfectants available nowadays. Many disinfectants of similar composition are sold under different trade names. Before buying a product with an unfamiliar name, compare types and values with a well-known product. Directions for dilutions given by the manufacturers should be closely followed. Continuous use of certain chemicals, particularly at inadequate concentrations, may produce a population of micro-organisms resistant to that chemical.

A brief description of some of the commonly used disinfectants follows:

1. Aldehydes

Glutaraldehyde and formaldehyde are the most commonly used disinfectant in this group. Glutaraldehyde is much stronger and more effective disinfectant than formaldehyde. It has a very wide range of activity and is a potent bacterial, virucidal, fungicidal, and sporicidal compound. It is also effective against both enveloped and non-enveloped viruses. It also has a fair residual activity and is effective in the presence of organic matter.

2. Formaldehyde

Formaldehyde is a gas. It is sold commercially in a 40% solution with water, under the name of formalin. Formalin is a very effective disinfectant, also cheap and easily available. It is used for fumigation of poultry house, brooder, and hatchery with potassium permanganate. Formaldehyde is usually generated by adding formalin to potassium permanganate in an earthen pot, or metal container. Because of the heat generated by the chemical reaction, glass containers should not be used. Take also steps to avoid risk of fire. The container should be deep and have a volume several times that of the combined chemicals, because a lot of bubbling takes place. Therefore, not more than 1 litre of formalin should be used per container. The container is placed in the room meant for disinfection. The ratio of formalin is about twice the amount of potassium permanganate. Potassium permanganate is poisonous. Therefore, both the compounds must be kept in accident-proof containers in a safe place.

About 60-70 g of potassium permanganate mixed with 120-150 ml of formalin is sufficient for disinfecting 100 cubic feet of space. Gas should be allowed to remain for 20-30 minutes in the rooms, incubators, brooders, etc. solution of formalin (5-10%) can be used for spraying a disinfectant for most bacteria and viruses. Usually a 4% solution is used. Formalin vapour is very good to disinfectant incubators, eggs, rooms, utensils, and is not very harmful except for its irritant action on eyes, nose, and skin.

Though formaldehyde is a powerful disinfectant, it has many disadvantages. It is extremely irritating to the conjunctiva and mucous membranes, and some people are very sensitive to it. Therefore, precautions must be taken to prevent its escape into areas, where people work. Operator should wear rubber gloves, when handling formalin. Its chief advantage is that formaldehyde can be used as a gas or vapour for fumigation of hatching eggs to destroy potential harmful shell contaminants, such as salmonella. It is a good disinfectant in the presence of some organic matter, and it does not insure equipment with which it comes in contact. Formaldehyde is also used to fumigate the inside of incubators and hatchers and their contents. Fumigation of incubators and eggs has been an established practice in the industry. The higher the humidity and temperature, the more effective is fumigation. Fumigation should not be done in incubators with eggs inside because of the danger of injuring embryos. 15 to 20 ml of pure formalin can disinfect about 100 cubic feet of a box or incubator.

Now the traditional method of formaldehyde fumigation is getting replaced by safer chemicals.

3. Phenols

Phenols are effective against bacteria, especially Gram-positive bacteria and enveloped viruses. They are bacteriostatic at lower concentration (i.e. stop the growth of bacteria but do not kill them) and bactericidal and fungicidal at higher concentration. Phenols are not effective against non-enveloped viruses and spores. Some commercial disinfectants have residual activity persisting after they have dried, giving continued suppression of bacterial and viral populations on sprayed surfaces. Therefore, they are effective in the presence of organic matter.

4. Chlorine compounds

Chlorine is bactericidal, virucidal, and fungicidal. However, it is relatively ineffective against spores. Its activity is reduced in the presence of organic matter, such as faeces and sol. Chlorine has poor residual activity.

5. Chlorinated Lime (Bleaching powder)

Chlorinated lime or bleaching powder, prepared by saturating slaked lime (i.e. lime treated with water) with chlorine gas, is one of the earliest recognised disinfectants. It has corrosive effect on metals and skin, and therefore, should be used cautiously after proper cleaning of floor. A 20% solution is used for disinfecting floor and utensils for feed and water. For water sanitization, use bleaching powder at the rate of 6 g per 1000 litres of water.

However, chlorinated lime has now been largely replaced by hypochlorites. If used according to directions, hypochlorites are highly efficient. Their main use is for egg washing and sanitizing, and for disinfecting incubators, incubator and Hatcher trays, small brooders, and water and feed containers. They can also be used on cement surfaces. All surfaces to be disinfected with hypochlorite solutions must first be thoroughly cleaned to ensure the greatest efficiency.

6. Organic Iodine Combinations

Iodine has long been recognised as an effective disinfectant. To overcome many of the disadvantages of the earlier products, **'iodophors'** have been prepared. The term **'iodophor'** refers to a combination of iodine with a solubilising agent that slowly liberated free iodine, when diluted with water.

A group of iodophors have been developed and are marketed for a wide variety of disinfectant uses. Some of these products have a built-in indicator of disinfectant activity. As the solution is used up, the normal amber (brownish-yellow) colour fades. When the solution is colourless, it is no longer effective. The product can be mixed in cold and hard water. They have a wide variety of uses. They can be applied safely to all surfaces, and are useful for disinfecting hatchery and incubator surfaces, incubator and hatchery trays, feeders, footwear, and poultry buildings. Iodophors are good disinfectants, but do not work well in the presence of organic matter. Like all other disinfectants, these compounds are most effective on clean surfaces. Iodophor has a broad disinfecting range, which includes bacteria, viruses, fungi and even coccidian and ova of parasites.

7. Quaternary Ammonium Surface Disinfectants

Quaternary ammonium products (quats) can be regarded as ammonium (NH4) compounds. Commercial products often contain various forms of ammonium chloride, or a combination of different ammonium compounds. Quaternary ammonium disinfectants are effective against bacteria, enveloped viruses, and some fungi. They are not effective against non-enveloped viruses and bacteria spores. However, they are moderately active in the presence of organic matter.

8. Copperhexidine

Although it is bactericidal, virucidal and fungicidal, it is effective against these agents than many other disinfectants. It is ineffective against non-enveloped viruses and spores.

9. Copper Sulphate

Copper sulphate is toxic to fungi. A 0.5% solution is generally used for destroying fungi on feed, hoppers, utensils, water fountains, and surrounding areas associated with outbreaks of fungal disease.

10. Lime

Lime is commonly used as a disinfectant for litter, floor, and poultry carcasses. It is mainly used in areas that are damp and cannot be exposed to the sun, as well as for disinfection of drains and faecal matter, and whitewashes. The action of lime depends on liberation of heat and oxygen, when the chemical comes in contact with water. Heat destroys bacteria and parasitic eggs and even coccidia, and keeps fungi under control. It should be applied liberally using at least 4-7 kg/100 feet^2. For disinfection of poultry manure, lime should be added at the rate of 90 kg/tonne of manure. It also disinfects wall and crevices, if a solution containing 38 parts lime and 15 parts sodium chloride is used for washing the wall. This combination acts as a good disinfectant. As lime has a caustic action, birds should be kept away from it, until it has become thoroughly dry.

11. Hot Water

Hot water adds to the efficiency of most disinfectants. If applied in the form of boiling water, it is effective without addition of any chemical.

12. Dry Heat

Dry heat in the form of a flame is effective, if the flame comes in contact with the ineffective agent to be killed. All methods involving direct flame are fire hazards, and not recommended except possibly on cement surfaces.

Table 1: Common disinfectants, concentration and method of use

Name	Concentration	Method of use	Approach surface for use	Remarks
Washing soda (Sodium carbonate)	3% solution in boiling water	Splashing, Rinsing utensils	Utensils & Floors	Little disinfection power but effective cleansing agent
Lime	½ kg lime/gallon of water as white wash + 5% phenol	Sprinkling dusting of powder of lime	Floors, walls and grounds	Use freshly prepared solution
Potassium permanganate	1:10,000 solution in water	Splashing	Floors, gutters and troughts	Disinfection action is due to oxidizing powder
Mercuric chloride	1 in 1000 parts of water	Splashing	Floors, gutters	Extremely poisonous, corrods metal, strong disinfectant

Phenol (carbolic acid)	2-5% solution in water	Splashing	Metallic objects and clothing	Good disinfectant
Formalin (40% formaldehyde)	5% solution in water 15-20 ml formalin + 15 gm of $KMNO_4$ per square meter space. 1 % solution in water	Splashing & fumigation	Houses internal atmosphere	Door and window must be opened before housing poultry
Silver nitrate	1% solution in water	Dissolution sprinkling	Eye infections	Too expensive to use in large amount
Copper sulphate	28 gms in 8000 gallons water	droops	Lakes reservoirs with ponds, plant	Useful to control algae and fungal growth
NaOH	2% for general use & 5% for splashing for killing spores	splashing	Floors, gutters equipment	Corrosive nature on metal, good cheaper disinfectant
Creosote	2-45 hot solution	splashing	Floor, gutter, wood trought	Less toxic and cheaper
Ethyl alcohol	70% solution in water	wiping	Skin, hands etc	Protect from flame
Iodine	2-5% solution in alcohol as tincture	wiping	Skin, wound, cuts etc	Very effective poisonous & irritating
Bleaching powder	30% available chlorine	dusting	Floor, gutter, passage	Protect from sunlight
Quaternary ammonium salts	1% solution	wiping	Udders, hands	Bactericidal more effective against gram+ than gram negative bacteria
Boric acid	5-6% solution	splashing	Skin, floor, walls, equipments, wounds	-

Mechanism of action

1. Destruction of bacterial cell or disruption of its organization.
2. Interference with energy utilization.
3. Interference with synthesis and growth.

Factor affecting germicidal action:

1. Concentration of disinfectant.
2. Time of exposure.
3. Temperature of disinfectant solution
4. Solution wheatear a fresh or stored.
5. Method of use brushing, spraying, sprinkling or dusting, etc.

6. Proper cleaning prior to disinfection to bring germs in close contact.
7. Kind of surface, mud, metal, wood, rubber, etc.

Functions of a disinfectant

1. Preparation of building: The various surfaces such as ceiling, walls, partitions and floors should be swept free of cobwebs, dust and dung. Any accumulation of filth must be removed by scrapping, scrubbing with a wire brush and warm water.
2. Selection of disinfectant: All factors that enter into evaluation of any disinfectant before a given compound is recommended are as follows:
   - Effectiveness- specific or general
   - Properties of solubility
   - Availability
   - Cost
   - Any additional preparation before use
   - Toxicity to tissues
   - Actions on metal wood, concrete floor, etc.
   - Stability of solutions
   - Odour, colour and actions on fabrics, etc.
3. Method of application of disinfectant: the solution should be applied rapidly in such a manner to cover entire surface requiring disinfection. On a limited surface, it may possibly be used with brush. For a large surface area, we may use sprayers with a spraying nozzle at the end.
4. Cautions : All disinfectants whether in form of dust or solutions are more or less poisonous and irritating to eyes, skin and respiratory passages. Persons applying these must be careful to avoid ingestion of these. Eyes, mouth and nose must be protected from dust. Goggles, gloves, respirator, etc. must be worm.

Cleanliness and Hygiene are the processes of adopting hygienic measures to nullify the factors, which deteriorate health and create conditions to secure health and ensures the production of good quality products.

Importance

Proper cleaning and sanitation remove most of germs and parasite along with dirt, thereby remaining germs are few in number and possibly in weakened condition so as to be harmless under ordinary conditions. Following are the main points in the context:

1. Proper sanitation discover causes of all preventable disease
2. Helps in providing most favourable conditions regarding water, air sheds, etc.
3. Helps in increasing the efficiency of animals
4. Helps in growth and development of animals, makes life vigorous and productive
5. Helps in minimizing contamination and good quality milk production
6. Helps dairy man to learn and make continuous efforts for improvement

Sanitation programme

i) Adequate ventilation

ii) Proper lighting

iii) Adequate drainage

iv) Proper cleaning

v) Proper disinfection

General points during cleaning and sanitation

1. Effective cleaning and disinfection is an essential component of good hygiene and thus, one of the key biosecurity measures for disease control. This should be carried out from time-to-time to reduce the build–up of pathogenic organisms and a disinfectant known to be effective against a large range of pathogens should be used regularly for prevention of ingress of the infection. It should address the disinfection of materials.
2. Approved disinfectants like chlorine dioxide and peracetic acid for disinfection or sterilization may be used.

3. Farm equipment entering the farm, cleanliness of personnel on the farm, disposal of dead birds and poultry manure and sanitizing the drinking water should be paid attention.
4. The area around poultry sheds should be kept clean from vegetation, food waste, plastic bottles, glass bottles, tins or drums.
5. Water testing should be done at regular intervals.
6. Proper ventilation with adequate air flow in all sheds is recommended.
7. Regular testing of Microbial load - at different places is recommended

Cleaning and disinfection of farm equipments

1. Feeding pans and drinking equipment used in the shed area should be kept clean daily.
2. Scrubbing should be done and then application of hot water followed by disinfection with an effective disinfectant.
3. Make sure all equipments that had contact with the poultry, lawn, garden and poultry equipments are washed and disinfected before taken to another place. The same should be followed, where some equipment are to be brought into the farm.
4. Keeping the shed equipments clean prevents pathogens from accumulating and causing health problems. Cages, if there, should be disinfected at regular intervals. They may be left in the sun and then they may be disinfected but it is essential to remove manure before disinfecting cages. Disinfectant will not work, if there is still manure present on items.
5. Newly purchased equipments should be thoroughly washed with soapy water or otherwise should be disinfected before use.
6. Newly purchased cages should also be subjected to washing with soapy water or should be disinfected.
7. Poultry equipments, such as egg crates, cages, shovels or rakes, should not be shared between family or neighbouring farms. Plastic or metal equipment may be preferred over wooden material.
8. Clean feeder and waterers daily.

Personnel hygiene

1. Specific over all clothing for employees must be provided.
2. Wash hands thoroughly before and after entering the farm area. Washing of hands can be done with soap or detergents with contact time of 10 minutes.
3. Wear clean clothes or coveralls while working with birds in the farm. The clothes should be washable with laundry detergent. Preferably for this purpose detergents or oxidizing agents (sodium hypochlorite dilute to give 2-3% available chlorine @ 2% with contact time of 10 minutes) and alkali (sodium hydroxide 2% solution or sodium carbonate anhydrous 4% solution with 10-30 minutes contact time) can be used, especially at the entrance on foot mats to clean the shoes gumboots and other items. Dirty clothes should be washed with detergent and hung out to dry in the sun. Quaternary-ammonium salts can be used for the treatment of walls, floors, ceilings and equipment, Cresolic-acid 2.2% solution or Synthetic phenols 2% solution can be used for the treatment of floors.
4. Since disease in poultry can be transmitted easily through boots, therefore, boots should be used after cleaning and disinfection. The best approach would be disinfecting footwear before and after working with birds or keeping a separate pair of shoes to work around birds and changing into other shoes, when leaving the premise. The person should use coveralls, which can be removed and cleaned, when leaving the premise. Boots should be washed in chlorinated water or with soapy water. Also, scrub boots while entering and existing.
5. When the care personnel needs to attend to chickens or other poultry (e.g. collecting eggs, feeding or watering, change of bedding or repair of fencing material), a change of clothes/ boots is required.
6. Medical check up of all workers coming in contact with livestock and feed should be done.

Cleaning and disinfection of poultry houses

After the post and pre-harvesting, the cleaning of shed is the first important and difficult part of bio-security. The house cleaning is mainly of two types according to birds harvested or remains:

i) Complete or terminal house cleaning : After removal of flock, this practices is considered. When flock has been harvested and removed completely, left feathers, droppings, letter and feed material and water, etc. removed. Then complete disinfection of the shed followed. Fumigate the poultry house firstly and then it should be subjected to an effective disinfection. Minimum 10 days waiting period is required before arrival of new flock of birds. To discourage the fungal growth, it should be ensured that no moisture content in house and litter before introducing the new crop of birds.

ii) Partial/concurrent house cleaning : This type of cleaning is required, when birds remain inside. This practice followed regularly according to schedule time.

- Clean the fans and windows.
- Sweep or clean the house from top to bottom.
- Remove the caked litter and wastes from the house.
- Place the clean litter in the house.
- Regularly disinfect the brooder guards, feeders, jugs, drinking water containers using iodophores and 5% sodium hypchlorite. Other chemical effective like sodium dodecyl sulphate, formalin and iodine compounds may also be used. Regularly sanitize the drinking water. For awareness and safety, disinfectant proportion used for cleaning must be displayed at the entrance of each shed/ hatchery.

Disinfection of Sheds and Comply with bio-security Procedures

Checklist for Implementing an Effective Poultry Bio-security Plan

Implementing any of these suggestions will reduce the risk of disease entry. Each additional step implemented will further reduce biosecurity risks.

1. Secure perimeter; Keep "restricted" signs posted at drive entrances
2. No trees or dense foliage around sheds, no roosting site for wild birds

3. Restrict entry to essential personnel and record entry.
4. Keep poultry houses locked; fasten from inside while inside.
5. Provide boots and coveralls for staff and visitors for each shed.
6. Staff should change into dedicated/disposable boots and coveralls upon entering each different shed. Clean footbaths may be appropriate within a shed, if changed regularly.
7. When caring for flocks, the resident flock manager should keep clothing (including shoes, boots, hat and gloves) separate from those worn off the farm.
8. After caring for the flock, change clothes completely and wash hands and arms before leaving premises.
9. Flock manager and other caretakers should not visit any other poultry flocks.
10. If possible, provide show facilities for visitors.
11. Remove poultry mortality daily. Store or dispose them off by an approved method.
12. Ensure staff and visitors are aware of the dangers of raising or visiting other avian species and their contact with your flock.
13. Essential visitors, such as owners, meter readers, service personnel, fuel and feed delivery drivers, and poultry catchers and haulers must wear protective outer clothing, including boots and headgear, before being allowed near the flocks.
14. Monitor vehicles entering premises for poultry pickup or delivery, feed delivery, fuel delivery, etc., to determine, if they have been scrubbed down and the undercarriage and tyres spray-disinfected before entering.
15. Minimize entry of equipment, supplies, etc. and take appropriate precautions, such as disinfection, removal from shipping boxes, etc.
16. Clean and disinfect all coops, crates and other poultry containers or equipment before and after use.
17. Maintain a strong vector control program for insect, mammalian and avian vectors. Maintain bait stations (bait stations must be numbered and a map kept of their location; bait stations must be

placed at regular intervals around the sheds), clean up feed spills, prevent entry by wild animals (rats, birds, insects) or pets (dogs, cats). Use screens in windows, air inlets, doors feed bin exhausts, etc.

18. Maintain minimal vegetation and no debris around poultry facilities to lessen food and shelter opportunities for vectors.
19. Ensure that feed, water and bedding sources are free from infectious agents.
20. Review your biosecurity plan and flock health program, including vaccination protocols, with veterinarian on a regular basis.
21. Sick or dying birds should be sent to a state laboratory for diagnosis. Commercial growers should contact their flock supervisor.

i) Movement restriction at poultry shed level

1. Keep the shed locked at all times.
2. Footwear dedicated for that shed, foot-dips and hand wash at entrance of every shed should be provided for. If felt necessary, farms may have higher norms, like having change room and shower facility even at shed level.
3. It should be ensured that all materials, drugs, vaccines, etc., are cleaned and disinfected and they should be have passed a quarantine storage period of 10 days in a especially designed storage room which should be cleaned regularly.
4. All material used in farm operations should be cleaned and disinfected before and after use.
5. Every shed should be provided foot dips at entrance and exit and it should be ensured that the dips are renewed on daily basis.
6. Fogging of the populated sheds should be a part of a prevention programme to minimize the risk of contamination. The disinfectant should be used with right dilution as per manufacture's direction.

ii) Restriction to visitors

1. Allow only essential people to contact the poultry kept in the farm.

2. Build a separate demonstration area and birds kept there should not later be stocked with shed-house birds.
3. If visitors have their birds of their own, do not allow them to come near to the birds.
4. Allow entry of the visitors in essential situation after taking all bio-security measures at farm entry as well after entry into the shed. These measures should include footbaths at the entry of farm and then at shed level, every visitor may change clothes/ cap/footwear, (go through shower-in policy, if required) and wear clean and disinfected clothes/ cap and boots. Specific coveralls and footwear for visitors are also to be provided.

iii) Restriction to farm workers

1. At the outset train the farm workers about the basic tenets of bio-security
2. Allow only the employees of that farm to handle the birds on a day-to-day basis.
3. Make sure that employees should not have a commercial or private bird operation, as they may transmit disease to the birds kept at the farm.
4. Do not allow farm workers to visit any other poultry farm or places where birds are kept. Similarly, the farm workers should not be allowed to visit the bird shows or bird fairs.
5. Workers engaged in rearing of one poultry species should not be allowed to visit other farms, where different poultry species is being reared.
6. All the farm workers should be allowed in the farm after going through all the biosecurity measures as mentioned for visitors.
7. All the farm workers must put off their clothes and boots after finishing their jobs and should go through shower-out policy.
8. All workers must wear clean and disinfected clothes during farm operations.
9. Frequent washing of hands with detergent or soap with sufficient contact time should be encouraged in day-to-day farm operations.

For set up the farm at the starting phases bio-security means i.e. Location and structural will be followed. For Operational bio-security programme, three main basic principles are:

- Isolation - The fencing should have to out of reach to other animals. The separation of flock on the basis of batches that can help to prevent them to contamination of diseases.
- Traffic control – Vehicle and transport system in the poultry farm managed and control properly. This should be properly clean and disinfected.
- Sanitation - Cleaning and disinfection are the component of sanitation. For hygiene and disease control, all the equipment, exposed surface, feeder, drinker, shed and cages go through this process.

Basic aspect of disinfection

Disinfection: It means act of destroying the cause of an infection. Since the causative agents of many diseases are extremely small and may remain indefinitely in dust, cracks and crevices of buildings disinfection must be carried out carefully to eradicate common enemies of life, such as bacterial, viruses, moulds and eggs of insects from contaminated premises.

Floor treatment : In some situations, it may be necessary to use floor treatments as well.

Table 2: Common floor chemical used for cleaning of floor

Compound	**Application Rate**		**Purpose**
	Kg/m2	Ibs/100ft^2	Kills Darking beetles
Boric Acid	As Necessary	As Necessary	Reduction of clostridium counts
Salt	0.25	5	Lowers PH
Sulphur Powder	0.01	2	
Lime(calcium oxide)	As Necessary	As Necessary	Disinfection

Table 3: Chemicals for sanitizing meat processing facilities

Compound Use	Concentration (ppm) *	Optimum use Temperature	Advantage	Disadvantage	Relative cost
Sodium hypochlorite	100 –200	Room temperature	Effective against a wide range of bacteria Corrosive, if not used	properly, organic matter reduces activity	+
Quaternary Ammonium Compounds	100 –200	Room temperature	Stable, long shelf life, less corrosive, additional cleaning properties	Leaves residues, high foaming, low efficiency on bacterial spores	++
Iodophor	25	Room temperature 35°C	Stable, long shelf life, less Corrosive	Can stain, less effective against bacterial spores	+++
Peroxyacetic acid	100 – 200	Chilled to room temperature	Effective against a wide range of organisms Peroxyacetic acid , biodegradable	Hazardous in concentrate form	++
Acid - anionic	200 – 400	Room temperature to hot	Less corrosive	Narrow spectrum of antimicrobial Activity	+++
Isopropyl alcohol	70% v/v	Room temperature	Fast acting	Not effective against spores, flammable	++

❑❑❑

Chapter **15**

Biosecurity

The word 'Biosecurity' consists of 'Bio' means life and 'security' means safety. Thus, bio-security implies safety of bird's life from diseases and disease causing organism. Biosecurity reduces mortality and morbidity.

When developing a biosecurity programme, following three components should be considered:

- Farm location : Farms should be located so that they are isolated from other poultry and livestock at least 3.2 Km (2miles) from the nearest poultry farm.
- Farm and house design : Housing should be designed to minimize traffic flow, to facilitate cleaning and disinfection. The house should be rodent proof with fencing around the farm. A clear and level area of 15m(50 ft) should extend right round the shed so that grass can be cut quickly and easily. An area of concrete or gravel extending to a width of 1-3m (3-10 ft) directly surrounding the house can discourage the entry of rodents and provide an area for washing and storing removable items .
- Operational procedures : Procedures must control the movement of people, feed, equipment and animals in the farm to prevent the introduction and spread of diseases. Routine procedures may be modified in the event of a change in disease status.

Biosecurity Programme

In a farm, the biosecurity programme is usually divided into following four important steps: (i) Security around the farm; (ii) Cleaning within the shed and around; (iii) Disinfection and (iv) Continuous disinfection programme.

The organic and inorganic dirt/debris in the poultry shed should be removed properly. The details of these programmes are linked with the structural and operational biosecurity measures for the sake of description.

a) Structural Biosecurity

The poultry farm should meet the following requirements:-

i) The perimeter of the site must be fenced and all opening must be secured leaving single door for entry and exit.

ii) A 2.13m perimeter around each shed/building must be kept free of all vegetations including trees; preferably be cemented.

iii) If the farm has multi-aged birds follow rigid contamination free movement of vehicle and man power.

iv) The drainage should be functioning especially where the soil is black or muddy with heavy rainfall.

v) All structural measures should be taken to prevent flies, rodent, and flying bird entry.

vi) Foot, vehicle dips and shower at the entrance are essential.

viii) Provide a close room near main gate for disinfection of any material coming from outside. Unload material in the room, fumigate with Formalin and Potassium Permanganate. Use 40 ml formalin (40 %) and 20g Potassium Permanganate ($KMnO_4$) for an area of m^3 (0.6 g $KMnO_4$ + 1.2 ml formalin for 1.0 ft^3). Add formalin to potassium permanganate in porcelain bowl kept inside the room (Caution- Never add potassium permanganate to formalin). Fumigate for 20 minutes and then ventilate the room through exhaust fan to allow formaldehyde gas to escape.

b) Operational Biosecurity

i) Broiler Units

a) It is difficult to follow biosecurity where live, culled birds are disposed off.

b) A disease surveillance/hygienic activities of water resources periodically be ensured to control bacterial & fungal load.

c) All in and all out system of management should strictly be followed.

d) A seven to ten days empty rest to shed is recommended for disinfectant to act.

e) Movement of birds among farms must be restricted.

f) Under threat of disease/infection scientific programme of disease detection, and diagnosis should be implemented.

ii) Layer Units

a) In large farms separate grower and layer unit at least 30 metres away should be located with the separate staff.

b) Appropriate vaccination programme/testing programme be ensured to protect flock against challenges and becoming carriers.

c) Since rodents are reservoir of salmonella, pasturella and even Mareks disease, hence their effective control is essential.

d) Care should be taken to monitor plastic tray hygiene if the plastic trays are exchanged while selling eggs to middle man. Egg vehicle should not be allowed inside the farm and delivery should be from a safe distance.

e) Post mortem facilities should be well-guarded.

f) In layer unit, the labours are provided with farm dresses especially chapels/shoes/apron to control entrance of infective agents.

g) Single door entry and exit with dress code are essential elements of a good hatchery.

Sources of Infection

Infections enter into a flock from various sources. To understand why various biosecurity measures are important, it is necessary first to examine briefly the sources and routes of infection. The survival time of various disease causing organisms varies from hours to months.

Table 1: Survival time of disease causing organisms

Disease	Infectious agent	Life-span away from birds
Ranikhet disease	Virus	Days to weeks
Gumboro	Virus	Months
Infectious bronchitis	Virus	Week to months
Infectious laryngotracheitis	Virus	Weeks
Avian influenza	Virus	Weeks to months
Marek's disease	Virus	Months
Lymphoid leukosis	Virus	A few hours
Fowl pox	Virus	Months to years
Infectious coryza	Bacterium	Hours to days
Salmonellosis	Bacterium	Weeks
Fowl cholera	Bacterium	weeks
Pullorum disease	Bacterium	Months
Fowl typhoid	Bacterium	Months
Staphylococcosis	Bacterium	Months
Avian tuberculosis	Bacterium	Years
Mycoplasmosis (MG, MS)	Mycoplasma	Hours to days
Coccidiosis	Protozoa	Months

1. Humans

Because of their movements, duties, curiosity, ignorance, lack of concern, carelessness, or total concentration on profits, humans constitute one of the greatest potential causes of introduction of disease. This is because they come in contact with infectious agents, use contaminated equipment, or manage their flocks in such a way that spread of disease is unavoidable.

Usually, foot wear (shoos, chapels) is suspected as the means of transport of disease, but hands can become contaminated with infected material, such as exudates (inflammatory fluids), when lesions and discharges are examined. Clothing can also become contaminated with dust, feathers, and droppings. At least one disease-causing organism (Ranikhet disease virus) has been found to survive for several days on the mucous membrane (i.e. lining) of the human respiratory tract, and has been isolated from the sputum.

2. Neighbours

A common source of infection is a disease outbreak at a neighbouring farm. Visits among poultry farmers are a common way of spreading diseases. If a neighbour's flock is infected with a serious disease, discuss it by telephone. It is best to warn neighbours not to visit, when disease is in progress, and certainly do not walk around on a neighbours farm for any purpose.

3. Contract workers/Labourers

Much of farm management requires periodic use of a group of workers for debeaking (beak trimming)., vaccination, blood testing, weighing, and shifting birds from one place to another. The farm manager usually has difficulty in finding workers who are easily available and have sufficient knowledge of handling poultry. Therefore, people who work hard at many poultry farms are contacted and hired. Such workers travel around the poultry farms handling many flocks, and must therefore, be regarded as a potential source of infection. The farm manager should take strict precautions to safeguard the health of every flock with which they work.

4. Visitors

No casual visitors are to be permitted in or near the poultry premises. Official visitors should always be taken to the flocks in increasing order of age, observing the precaution that they have not visited any other farm on that day. They should be provided with footwear and a clean outfit of clothing before visiting the flocks. Visitor's vehicles should not be allowed inside the farm premises.

Disease outbreaks on a farm have been known to follow the visit of a careless visitor. If visitors do not enter premises or buildings, they cannot bring in or carry away diseases.

The source of a new or dreaded disease like Gumboro is often puzzling. World trade and travel are becoming more common place. It is not uncommon for a person to leave one farm in the morning and be visiting another farm or place of business in another part of the country on the same day. Some disease agents easily survive during that period. All who travel should be aware of this, and must be careful against introducing the disease into their own flocks, or into the premises of friends, or fellow farmers, when returning from a trip.

5. Recovered Carriers

Carrier birds are those which appear to have recovered from disease, but still retain the infectious organism in some part of the body. While they appear healthy, the infectious organism continues to multiply (increase in number) in the body and to be shed into the environment. Like actively infected flocks, they can spread a disease on a farm and thus, constitute a threat to other birds. Many commonly occurring diseases are known to be transmitted by carriers.

6. Multiple Ages

Multiple ages on premises constitute a serious disease threat, from both diseased bird and recovered carriers. This is particularly important, if birds of different age groups are closely associated through management practices, or nearness. Disease organisms from sick birds, or recovered carriers, are passed by various ways, including direct contact, to each new susceptible flock brought into the premises. Serious drops in production may occur in young laying flocks moved into laying premises, where carrier birds from previous disease outbreaks had remained.

7. Induced-Moulted Hens

Induced-moulting of laying hens (or brooders) is usually practised, particularly during times of economic stress to meet an emergency egg demand, or improve declining shell quality, or because it is considered economical at that time. One advantage of keeping induced-moulted hens, rather than rearing new replacement growers, is that old hens are not likely to suffer from a disease that normally occurs during the rearing age. If such flocks are moulted and kept in the same house, then there is no risk of disease problems developing. On the other hand, a farmer who collects spent hens for moulting from many poultry farms and mixes them on one premise at one time runs a serious risk. This is because any of the moulted groups may be carriers of a disease to which the others are susceptible.

8. Poultry Show Birds

Birds exhibited at poultry shows may be exposed to infected or symptomless carrier birds of exhibitors from which they contract disease. The contact-infected birds may not develop symptoms until returned to the owner's farm, where they may then be a source of new infection. A basic rule for show birds is that they should never be returned to the owner's farm. If birds must be shown, such should be selected that can be sold after the exhibition. If the birds must be returned, they should be quarantined for several weeks.

9. Mixed Species of Poultry

One species which is naturally very resistant to a disease may act as a carrier of that disease for another species that is very susceptible. For example, histomoniasis may cause mild death losses in chickens, but in turkey, the losses can be extremely serious. Also, a silent mycoplasma infection in chickens may spread to mycoplasma-free turkeys and result in extremely serious sinusitis and air sac infection. Therefore, two species should never be run together.

Some diseases may be rather harmless in one species of chicken, but very serious in another. Also, keep meat and laying chickens separate, since the same disease may have different economic importance in the two types.

10. Hospital Pen

Sick birds from several pens collected into one hospital pen, or house, and later returned to their respective pens may carry back one or more diseases contracted while in the hospital area. Therefore, hospital pens are not recommended for routine segregation of sick birds unless they are ultimately to be sent to the diagnostic laboratory, or burned. If used for a special purpose (such as observation, injury, pecking), there should be a temporary arrangement within the house, and it should hold birds from only one pen or house.

11. Backyard and Pet Fowl

Poultry kept as pets, or to supply household eggs or meat, are just as capable of carrying and transmitting diseases as are commercial flocks.

12. Soiled Vehicles and Equipment

Diseases and parasites can be carried on vehicles and equipment. Vehicles and equipment usually have accumulations of litter and faeces that can be a threat to other farms and houses. Soiled vehicles and equipment can carry disease organisms. They should be washed free of litter and droppings, and also disinfected after each transport of live birds, before use in another farm area. One gram of chicken faeces can contain enough virus particles to infect one million (ten lakhs) birds with avian influenza.

Fowl pox, Gumbroo disease and Marek's disease viruses, coccidian, roundworm eggs, and other infectious material can be carried on crates (large containers for carrying eggs and birds), footwear, and vehicles, particularly on the floor and foot control pedals of a vehicle.

Artificial insemination equipment, particularly reused inseminating tubes, offer an excellent method of transmitting disease.

Poultry transporting vehicles and equipment can spread infectious material through feathers, faeces, blood, exudates, an skin scabs (crusts) left in the creates, or picked up after use before being taken to another farm.

13. Laboratory exposure

A famer, particularly a small flock owner, may like to take a bird home after a veterinarian has examined it at the laboratory. While in the laboratory, even for a short time, live birds have a good chance to contract some infectious agent. Therefore, no bird should be returned from the laboratory to the farm, because it could develop disease and be the source of a new infection on the home premises. The bird should be sacrificed and subjected to post-mortem.

A disease may be carried from laboratory to a farm by careless laboratory to a farm by careless laboratory or service workers, or the farmers. Therefore, precautions against carrying disease from the laboratory to the farm should be taken by the farmer and service worker.

14. Rodents

Rodents are a group of small animals with strong sharp front teeth, such as rats, mice, squirrels and beavers (see "rodents"). Rodents contaminate feed and litter with their faeces. They are particularly important in the control of Salmonella, because they are frequently infected with these organisms and can maintain and spread the disease on a farm.

15. Household Pets

Dogs and cats, like rodents, are capable of harbouring enteric organisms (i.e. those infecting intestine) which are infectious to poultry. When these pets are not confined to the household area, but roam among the poultry in the pens and farms, they constitute a serious health hazard. Such pets are just as capable of carrying contaminated material on their feet and in their hair, as people.

16. Wild Birds

Wild birds are capable of carrying a number of diseases and parasites. Some cause illness in the wild birds themselves; for others, the birds act as mechanical carriers. Every effort should be made to prevent their nesting in the poultry farms. Domestic pigeons can also be a source of dangerous strains of Ranikhet disease virus.

17. Insects

Many insects act as transmitters of disease. Some are intermediate hosts for blood and intestinal parasites; others are mechanical carriers of disease through their biting parts. Still others, because of their feeding habits and hiding places, appear to be reservoirs of disease by means of which the infectious agent survives from one flock to the next.

18. Feed

Some ingredients may contain infectious agents, particularly Salmonella, from contamination at their source, or anywhere along the production line, or storage areas. Pelleting, if done properly, is a practical method of greatly reducing infectious agents because of the heat generated in the process. Meat meal and bone meal are the feed ingredients most likely to introduce Salmonella species. The risk can be avoided by using only vegetable protein ingredients, supplemented, as necessary with synthetic amino acids.

Management Factors in Disease Prevention

Good disease-prevention practices have been compared with a chain, which is only as strong as its weakest link. Many sound principles may become worthless from failures to carry out one or two related ones, which are either ignored or not considered essential. Although, it may not always be possible to use all the practices, the more are followed, the greater are the chances of avoiding disease outbreaks.

1. Isolation

It is very important that the poultry farm has an isolated location. This will avoid most disease problems. No exact minimum distance from other poultry farms can be stated because this is influenced by prevailing winds, climate, type of houses, and other factors. The greater the distance from other poultry farms, the less chances of contracting disease from them. Isolation can be achieved by taking advantage of natural or artificial barriers, such as rivers, creeks, hills, cities, towns, or forests.

Not all farmers follow the same disease control practices. A close neighbour may ignore them and is then burdened with diseases until forced out of business by economic pressures. In the meanwhile, disease organisms present on his farm may be spread by air, or carried by various vectors (i.e. organisms, such as insects that transmit disease) and formites (inanimate substances that mechanically spread disease-producing organisms) to neighbouring farms. Thus, a disease sometimes may enter into even well-managed farms. Until s disease has been eradicated, it serves as a reservoir and potential source of infection for future flocks on the same premises and also those on the neighbouring p remises. The closer the houses of one premises to those of another, the more likely is the spread of infection to healthy birds on a neighbouring farm. Farmers who do not minimize losses, go out of business. Many left out poultry farms are purchased or leased by other poultry farmers.

2. Birds of One Age at One Farm

From disease prevention point of view, it is always better to have birds of only one age at one farm, rather than having birds of different ages. When birds of one age are maintained, houses become vacant each time growers are moved to the layer premises, or each time the broilers are sold, or each time the old layers are sent to market. The premises are then cleaned, washed, and disinfected, and led to vacant for as long as possible, but at least for two weeks before healthy stock is introduced.

Keeping premises vacant is most effective in controlling disease organisms which do not survive for long outside the bird. This applies to most respiratory infections (mycoplasma infection, infectious coryza, laryngotracheitis). However,, it is not much effective in controlling disease agents that are more resistant and survive long periods in nature (coccidian, cloastridia). In general, the longer poultry house remains vacant, the lower the number of surviving disease-producing organisms.

Moreover, in birds of one age at one farm, should a disease occur, the flock can be treated and handled in the best way possible until its disposal. All this is not possible, when birds of different ages exist on a farm.

The best way to prevent infection from carrier birds is to remove the entire flock from the farm before any new replacements are added, and to rear young stock in complete isolation from older recovered birds on a separate segment of the farm, or preferably on another farm and in an isolated area.

3. Functional Units

For certain economic reasons, it is not always possible to limit the entire farm to a single age of poultry. In such cases, it should be divided into spate units, or areas for different groups of birds. Each area is then periodically kept vacant, cleaned, and disinfected. Much stricter security procedures for personnel, bird and equipment movements are necessary for this type of operation. There is no definite formula for minimum distances between houses or units. The most important factor in dividing the farm into isolated units is to provide units that can be quarantined (kept in isolation) to prevent spread and facilitate elimination of disease, should it occur.

4. Building Construction

The first rule in poultry house construction is to prevent flying wild birds and insects from entering. This is because many carry mites and harbour them on their nests. Also, many species of wild birds have been found susceptible to some common viral and bacterial diseases of poultry, and thus, could at as carriers. Bird-proofing can be done in open-type houses in hot climates.

a) Entrances

An area (a slope or ramp) of concrete at the entrance of poultry house helps in preventing entry of disease into the unit. Rain and sunshine keep the area clean and sterilized. A water tap, boot brush, and covered metal container of disinfectant should be made available on the slope for disinfecting footwear (shoes, 'chappals', etc.) This further helps in keeping litter and soil-borne diseases out of the houses. Shoes must be thoroughly cleaned before the person steps into the container of disinfectant. Failure to remove organic matter will prevent even the strongest of disinfectants from destroying disease-producing organisms. Moreover, the disinfectant is infective unless replaced frequently to ensure a potent solution at all times.

b) Ventilation

Poultry buildings should be constructed to provide protection against violent or severe weather conditions, yet not create stress conditions, such as excess dust, insufficient ventilation with ammonia build-up (a gradual increase), or wet litter.

There are many advantages of windowless and temperature-controlled (i.e. environmentally controlled) houses, but one serious drawback is the development, in some cases, of extremely dry and dusty litter. Collibacillosis outbreaks are usually associated with inhalation of excessive dust. Coccidal oocyts require moisture to develop into the infective stage. Extremely dry litter prevents their development. On the other hand, improper ventilation can lead to excessively wet litter, which favours the survival and development of coccidian and other parasites.

Ammonia fumes develop in wet litter. If ventilation is poor and fumes accumulate, they may reach high concentration to prevent growth and performance of birds, cause kerato-conjunctivitis, and aggravate respiratory infections.

Litter will dry better, if it can be stirred (mixed up) frequently. However, in spite of all efforts, it may remain wet in winter or in humid climates, if wetness and excess ammonia concentration persist, litter should be replaced and ventilation improved.

c) Floors and Cages

All surfaces inside the building should be impervious material (i.e. not allowing water to pass through), such as concrete, so that it can be thoroughly washed and disinfected.

Raised slatted floors have been used successfully for years for laying chickens, both for adults and rearing birds. Such floors have alternated wooden pieced and spaces, each about ¾ inch wide, to allow droppings to fall through the open spaces and be out of reach of the birds. This prevents recycling of infection and thus, helped in the control of intestinal diseases and parasites. Coccidial infection is thus avoided or greatly reduced. Broilers are likely to develop leg problems and breast blisters, if raised on completely slatted or wire floors.

Keeping laying hens in cages has become an accepted practice in both closed and open-type houses in hot climates. Cages and wire floors are widely used also to rear growers, destined for cages as adults. The system is so successful in preventing intestinal diseases that birds have no chance to develop immunity to them. Coccidiosis occurs, if chickens reared in cages are transferred to litter floors. Drugs can be used successfully to control coccidiosis in these birds.

d) Feeders and Drinkers

Rats, mice and other rodents should be out of feed because they may introduce and spread salmonella, or other disease organisms, which can be the source of an outbreak in the poultry flock.

Feed spilled in litter increases intake of litter and litter-borne disease agents. For example, more coccidial oocyts and less coccidostat are ingested, and a clinical disease may occur. If poultry are allowed to eat litter, mortality and depression can occur from impaction of the gizzard, and litter fragments may cause enteritis by mechanical irritation.

Feed troughs should have some type of guard to keep poultry out, and should not be overfilled to avoid spilling of feed into litter. Feeders without guards allow defecation into feed, which results in the spread of infectious agents shed in faeces. Wet feed in litter attracts wild birds and rodents and provides a good medium for growth of fungus and moulds, which can cause liver, kidney, immune system disorder, or other damage to poultry.

Drinkers are usually set or hung over the litter area. In such a case, drinkers should be so managed that the spillage of water on the litter is minimum. Drinkers are basically of two types: (1) those which provide a constant reservoir of water, such as troughs i.e. channels and hanging plastic bells, and (2) nipple drinkers, which supply water on demand, when activated by a bird.

Drinkers which provide an open reservoir of water must be cleaned and disinfected regularly to prevent the build-up of potentially disease-causing organisms in the water supply. These drinkers are also more prone to spillage and may cause problems of wet litter. The advantages of nipple drinkers are that they provide water free of organisms which are commonly present in the poultry houses, and also there is a decreased water spillage. The dry litter conditions provided by nipple drinker's result in decreased growth or maturation of coccidian, bacteria, and fungi in the litter.

e) Feed and Water Medication

In spite of all precautions, birds may become sick. When birds are grouped in large numbers in one big pen, separation and treatment of individuals is not possible; mass medication and vaccination are then necessary, if any treatment is to be given.

Feed medication is not the best method of treatment for sick birds because of the loss of appetite (desire for food) and their inability to compete for feed. Water medication is better because the sick birds usually drink, when they will not eat. Mass medication keeps the disease in check until the bird can respond with a successful immune response. Mass vaccination through drinking water is an accepted and successful labour-saving practice. If drinking water is chlorinated or otherwise treated, the sanitizing agent may destroy the vaccine. Therefore, use untreated or distilled water for mixing and administering water vaccine.

Several methods are used to reduce, remove, or neutralise chlorine in chlorinated water supplies. The best practical method is to add protein to the water, when mixing vaccines. A common practice is to add 1 lb of non-fat dried milk to 50 gallon water, in tanks.

If a building is constructed with a big water tank, the tank should be of plastic, or lined with some non-reactive protective substance, and should be easy to reach for cleaning and for mixing of medicines. A metering device to measure feed and water consumption is useful to keep track of the health of the flock. Use of a watering system with nipple drinkers for individual cage units helps in preventing spread of disease.

Personnel Control

1. Company and Farm Workers

Managers, supervisors, and owners are sometimes the worst people to break the sanitation rules. These people usually visit many different types of poultry farms, farm units, poultry industries, and spread disease organisms. They should set a good example for the workers. One of the most important aspects of disease control is awareness on the part of everyone, that is, managers, supervisors, owners, workers, feed and supply delivery people; egg, bird and litter transporters; and all those who visit or work on poultry farms, that each has an important role in the disease-prevention programme.

2. Visitors

Visitors can cause only minimum harm, if they cooperate fully with strict sanitary rules. When they enter the poultry premises (houses, sheds), it is important that they wear disinfected rubber overshoes (gumboots) and other footwear. Also, they should wear protective clothes, such as clean aprons. Disposable plastic boots may become punctured, when used on gravel (mixture of small stones and coarse sand), or other sharp surfaces. Therefore, only heavy plastic disposable boots should be used. These sanitary precautions are particularly essential, when entering brooding and rearing houses, but will be helpful in keeping disease out of any house or pen.

Sanitary Environments

A) Grounds around the Buildings

1. Rodent Control

Heaps of rubbish and unused equipment are good hiding and breeding places for rats, mice and ground squirrels (see 'rodents'). These may serve as reservoirs of disease and contaminate troughs (water channels) with their faeces. Rodents are reluctant to travel over open spaces which do not provide protective cover. A 20- metres strip (belt) of shortly cut grass, or gravel, discourages the migration of rodents into the poultry building from surrounding areas. It is more difficult to get rid of rodents once the premises are infected, than to keep them out from the beginning.

2. Insect Control

Many parasites and disease agents are: (1) harboured from one generation to another in insects, e.g., Marek's disease, or (2) require an insect for an intermediate stage of development e.g., tapeworms, or (3) are simply carried from bird to bird mechanically or by biting, e.g., fowl pox virus. Control measures against insects are a part of the sanitary environment and clean-up.

Spraying the area around building with an insecticide prevents insect build-up. A good practice during cleaning is to spray the grounds, litter, and buildings with an insecticide immediately after removal of the birds. Then allow a few days for effective insect killing before removing litter for cleaning and disinfection. After cleaning, the building should be sprayed again with an insecticide to prevent re-infestation.

B) Disposal of Dead Birds

Dead birds disposal have become a major problem in poultry industry. This is because farms have become larger and some of the older methods of disposal are no longer environmentally acceptable. Following precautions must be observed in the disposal of dead birds:

1. Dead birds must be removed from the cages and the poultry house daily.
2. Keep the containers having dead birds covered at all times to prevent contact with flies and other insects, dogs, cats, and free-flying birds.
3. After dead birds are handled, wash your hands, and disinfect the house and its equipment.
4. Don't allow trucks or people picking up dead birds to visit any area on the farm.
5. The disposal pits should be in an isolated area of the farm.

Foci of Infection

When birds die from infectious diseases, carcasses remain a source of infection for other birds on the same or other farms. Also, sick birds discharge infectious material into the environment and should be removed from the flock and killed in a manner that will not allow the discharge of blood or exudates. Whatever the cause, all carcasses should be disposed off by one of the following methods to prevent spread of disease:

1. Burning

Burning is the most reliable way of destroying infectious material. Many smokeless, odourless incinerators for disposal of animal carcasses are available commercially.

2. Burying

Where environmental regulations allow, a deep pit may be dug and the carcasses buried so that animals cannot get at them. The best and easiest way is to use a backhoe (an excavating machine) and dig a deep narrow trench (a long narrow channel, a ditch). Each day's collection of dead birds can be deposited and covered until the trench is filled.

3. Pit or Tank Disposal

For small losses, a decomposition pit can be used. Precautions should be taken to ensure that: (1) it is not located where it will contaminate drinking water supplies, (2) that walls will not collapse, (3) that animals will not dig into it, (4) that flies or other insects cannot get into it, and above all, (5) that children cannot fall into it. The pit cover should be sealed with tar paper or plastic, and be strong enough to hold a foot of soil on it.

4. Cooking

Freshly dead birds can be rendered (i.e. treated to convert) into fertilizer or other products. The rendering temperature should be adequate for sterilisation. It should be remembered that commercial or contract transporters of dead carcasses can introduce another disease from some other outbreak, unless strict precautions are taken.

5. Composting

Composting is the process by which a mixture of decayed organic matter is converted into fertiliser. Composting of poultry carcasses is an important method of disposal. Compost mixtures of straw, whole poultry carcasses, manure, and water in the proportions of 1:1:1:5:0.5, respectively (one third of water added to each layer), decompose rapidly and odourlessly. Composts heat rapidly, reach temperatures of between 145° and 165°F, and reduce soft tissues completely within 14 days. The process is biologically reliable. Escherichia coli, Salmonelle-like bacteria, and Gumboro virusget destroyed.

C) Buildings and Runs

1. Clean Buildings

A clean hygienic environment is good protection against disease outbreaks.

2. Litter Removal

When all the birds from a house are disposed off and the house falls vacant, the litter or droppings should be removed before cleaning. With very big poultry farms, proper and economical disposal of litter and poultry manure has become a serious problem. There is no clear-cut answer. Generally, it is removed far away from the buildings so that insects do not crawl or fly back into houses; and to dry it, compost it, or spread it onto fields and work it into the soil. If cleaning is done while chickens are still present, remember that hired people, trucks and equipment may recently have been on another farm, where a disease may have occurred.

For most disease agents, composting of litter or droppings is sufficient, because of the heat generated. However, one must remember that whatever litter is spilled or piled, it remains as a disease reservoir for varying lengths of time.

3. Washing and Disinfection

Once the litter or cage droppings have been removed, drinkers, egg collecting and other equipment, walls, floors, cages, outside concrete runs, and entries to buildings should be washed thoroughly and disinfected. If the supply of water is limited and washing is not possible, dry cleaning may be sufficient, if it is thorough, and includes scraping and sweeping or vacuuming surfaces, corners, ledges, nests, and feeders. The amount of disinfectant used on dry-clean surfaces must be increased over that required for washed surfaces.

If possible, it is better to clean the house without removing equipment. If not, all portable equipment should be removed, soaked with water, then thoroughly washed and dried. A high-pressure water hose is effective. Equipment that cannot be removed should be washed in place, and then the entire inside building surface washed clean.

After washing, disinfection should be done (see chapter 30: 'Disinfection'). There are many good disinfectants sold under different trade names. Follow the manufacturer's recommendations. The important thing is that the surfaces be clean before application. Disinfectant applied on dirt-covered surfaces be clean before application. Disinfectants applied on dirt-covered surfaces are ineffective and washed. Not only are they inactivated by organic material in the dirt, but they never reach the infectious organisms below it. Thorough washing removes most infectious agents from the house and equipment, and leaves a clean surface, so the disinfectant can reach those that remain. Two or four weeks of vacancy (resting) before a new flock is moved in, is additional protection against carrying over of diseases. However, the vacancy period (downtime) should be taken only as an additional measure, and not as a substitute for thorough cleaning, washing, and disinfection.

4. Built-up Litter and Un-cleaned Buildings

Farmers demand hicks are free of infectious agents acquired through egg transmission, or from unsanitary hatchery or delivery environments. To maintain this standard, these healthy new flocks should be placed in cleaned and disinfected buildings, with fresh clean litter. To provide these, ideal conditions is expensive because of labour and litter costs. Also, suitable litter materials are becoming less available. To reduce production costs and cope with shortages, rearing of several successive flocks on the same (built-up) litter has become an economically acceptable practice with broilers, where the life-span is very short and birds of one age group in each farm permit their complete removal at the end of each lot.

In developed countries, this trend has become common with the use of litter processing machinery, which can be break up caked litter and produce a litter that is acceptable. However, the continual re-use of such built-up litter will result in an increase in the numbers of infectious organisms and parasites within the litter.

The practice of re-using litter is not advisable for rearing layer flocks, where the life-span is usually more than 18 months. In any case, those who re-use litter should be fully aware of the possible risks involved, and should follow other sound disease control practices to minimize the dangers.

If old litter be re-used, remove any caked or excessively dirty litter, accumulated feathers, and decomposed carcasses. A layer of fresh clean litter should then be placed under the heating brooders and over the area where the young will be confined, or will spend most of their time (i.e. the first few weeks of their life). One disadvantage of multiple brooding on the same litter is the excessive dust that accumulates. Inhalation of the dust provides a means of entry into the respiratory tract for bacterial and fungal spores.

Rodent & Pest Control in Poultry Sheds

a) The poultry house and its surroundings are ideal places for rodents, such as rats, mice, mongoose, squirrels due to availability of feed and hiding places. Rodent causes enormous damage to building and also financial losses.

Damage Caused by Rodents

i) Eat considerable quantity of feed (10-113 gm/day) and also spoils it by defecation and urination.

ii) Burrow holes under floor and make pathways for movement.

iii) Carry poultry infection by acting as carrier of *E. coli*, Mareks, etc.

iv) Rat kills and causes injury to weak chicks. A single mongoose will not only kill chick but kill adult caged birds also.

v) Rodent movement in night causes panic effecting performance of flock.

Control Measures

i) Construct a rat proof shed.

ii) Repair holes on floor, damage roof, walls & chicken mash, etc. promptly.

iii) Avoid extra storage of feed in the shed as easy excess to rodents.

iv) Use rodenticides periodically to keep check on their population.

v) Use rat traps and facilities provided by government on rat control.

vi) Remove dead bird quickly else rodent may become carnivores.

b. Pest is an important mechanical vector of many human and poultry diseases. The most common species encountered in poultry operations is house-fly (*Musca domestica*) . This fly breeds in moist, decaying plant material, spilled feed, waste egg material, wet manure and in cracks and crevices. Eggs hatch into white, cylindrical larvae (maggots) in 12 to 24 hours.

Control Measures

i) Dry manure management is highly effective in reducing pest populations. Eggs are laid on breeding media like manure hatch out in moist or wet material, where they remain until ready to pupate.

ii) Water management with respect to the moisture content of manure is important for effective pest control.

iii) Quickly remove dead birds and broken eggs.

iv) Clean up and dispose off feed spillage immediately.

v) Treat the flock for diarrhoea.

vi) Avoid high salt content in the feed which may lead to increased water consumption as well as wet droppings.

vii) Mechanical Control of Pests : Mechanical control can be accomplished through the use of various types of pest traps, electrically operated insects killer (pest ban, pest killers) and mechanical burning. Mechanical burning of flies in their resting areas like chain link mesh, trashes, etc. may be helpful to reduce adult pest population.

viii) Chemical Control of Pests : Chemical control consists of the application of insecticides and should always be considered supplemental to sanitation, management options to control pests. Rotational use of variety of different classes or group families of insecticides or pesticides can minimize the chances of developing chemical resistance.

❑❑❑

Chapter 16

Processing and Preservation of Eggs

With increasing urbanization, eggs and live birds needs to be packed and transported in good condition to distant places and distributed through retail outlets to consumers. Though we think that, it is very simple and easy to transport eggs and live poultry birds, you should keep in mind that these live birds are very sensitive and the eggs are easily breakable and spoil quickly, if not stored and transported properly. Hence, they should be handled, packed, stored and transported properly. You will be surprised to know that, only 10 % eggs and 30% broilers are sold as processed product in our country and the remaining are sold without further processing. Therefore, the predominant modes of disposal of chicken in the market are by sale of live bird at the farm and slaughter at retail poultry meat shops. The tasks involved in marketing of eggs include collecting, sorting and grading; packaging on farm or transporting to a grading, packaging and processing plant; storing; moving through wholesale and retail channels; and selling directly or indirectly to consumers.

Harvesting and Post-harvesting of Eggs

Though, management of laying birds like feeding, care and managements etc. are very important activities in a layer farm, harvesting (collection of eggs) and post-harvest activities like handling, storage, packaging and transportation of eggs are equally important for the overall economics of the farm. This section will deal with the egg harvesting and post-harvest activities in a layer farm.

Collection and Handling of eggs

Collection of eggs is one of the major activities in a layer farm since , eggs are the major end product. Since eggs are fragile in nature and can break easily with slight application of pressure, it is necessary to know how to handle eggs during its collection, sorting/grading, storage, packaging and transportation. The points to be kept in mind during collection and handling of eggs are as follows:

- ***Method of collection :*** In case of small to medium sized layer farms, eggs are generally collected manually (by hand). However, in large layer farms, it is suggested to use automatic egg collection equipment in order to save time, cost and labour.

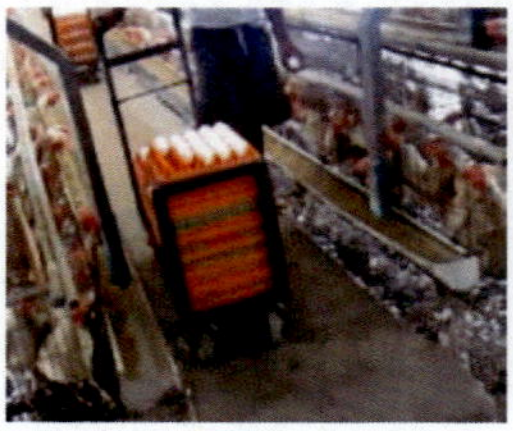

Manual Egg Collection

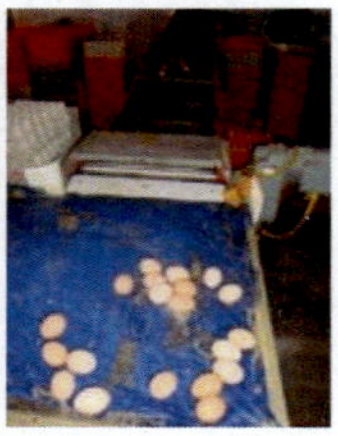

Automatic Egg Collection Equipment

Methods of Egg Collection

- Frequency of eggs : Eggs should be collected twice in a day. Eggs are generally collected in the morning and afternoon. Care should be taken to maintain a time schedule for collection of eggs in order to save time and labour.
- Equipment/tools/utensil : Always collect eggs in an easy to clean and disinfect containers like coated wire baskets or plastic containers. Avoid using metal containers, as they are difficult to clean and there are chances of staining eggs from rusted metal and contamination from other materials. Eggs can also be collected directly into the plastic or wood pulp egg filler flats/ trays.
- The person collecting eggs should be clean, healthy and in hygienic conditions.
- Collection : Collect clean, hygienic and unbroken eggs separately. Dirty, soiled and broken eggs should be collected separately to avoid cross-contamination.

Clean, hygienic and unbroken egg

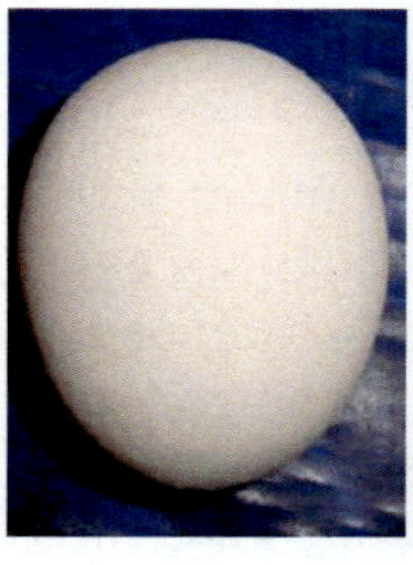

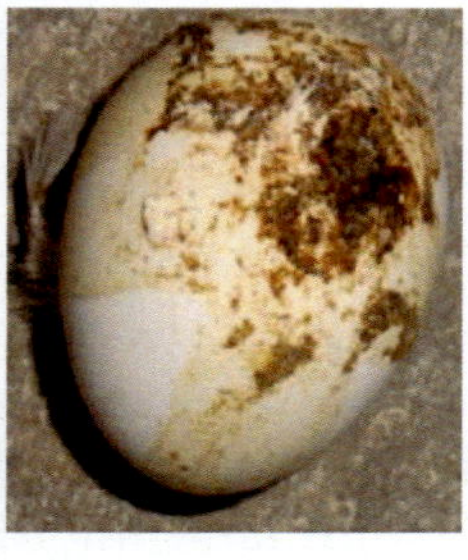

Dirty and soiled egg

- Defective (Thin shelled, mis-shapen, etc.) or broken/cracked eggs should not be stored and should be discarded immediately.

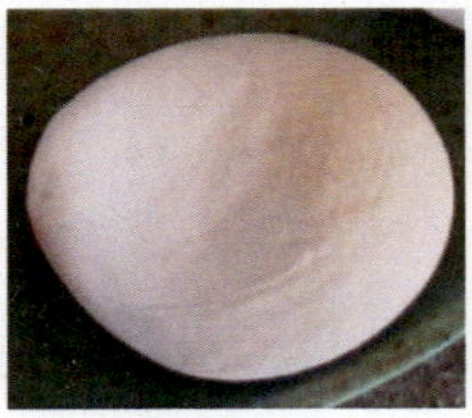

Mis-shapen eggs

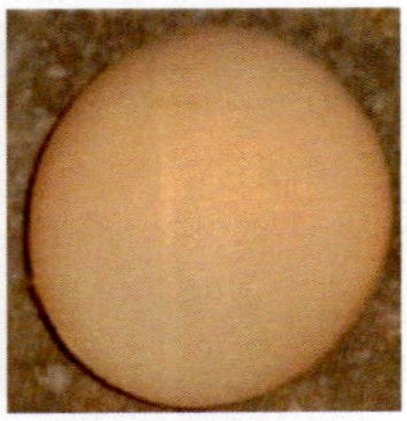

Thin-shelled egg

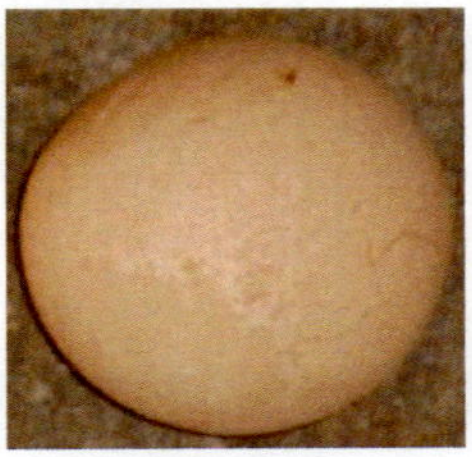

Shell-less egg

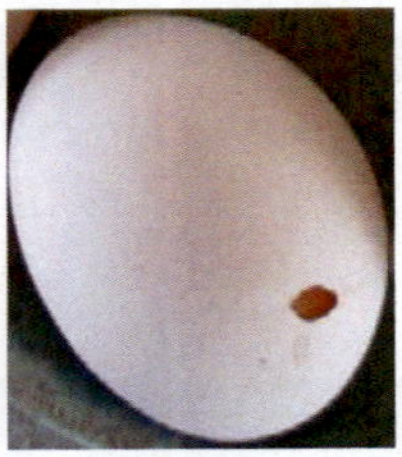

Shell-less egg

Defective and broken eggs

- ***Handling eggs :*** Eggs should be handled gently,and very carefully while collecting from the laying cages or from the Nest-box or floor of layer house.
- ***Egg cleaning :*** Eggs which are clean fetch better prices. Therefore, any feather or dirt sticking to the egg should be removed gently without damaging egg coating. It is not advisable to wash the dirty eggs, as it will remove natural protective coating and may help in the entry of harmful microbes into the egg through tiny pores present in the egg shell. Excessively dirty eggs should not be cleaned and must be discarded immediately to prevent cross-contamination.

Sorting and Grading of Eggs

Different size and weight eggs fetch different prices. Therefore, eggs should be sorted and graded before marketing to get better price:

a) ***Sorting :*** It is a common practice to sort eggs before storing or selling. Eggs can be manually sorted based on the size or weight.

b) ***Grading :*** Eggs should be graded before packaging or storage based on weight, shell colour & thickness, and interior egg quality. Commercially, grading of egg is an important step to assess the quality of product for fetching best price and shelf life (storage stability). Grading is universally accepted and considered useful in marketing of any product. Normally, larger eggs fetch better price than smaller eggs. Similarly, dark yellow coloured yolk is always preferable than the dull or light yellow coloured yolk. Brown egg shells are preferred over white colour.

The best and easiest way of grading eggs is by candling using a candler. Candler is a small electric tool which produces a beam of light, which when passed through the egg in dark environment helps to get an idea about the internal quality of eggs without breaking open. It is used to remove defective eggs by easy identification of cracks in the shell and other defects like blood spots, meat spots, etc. inside the egg.

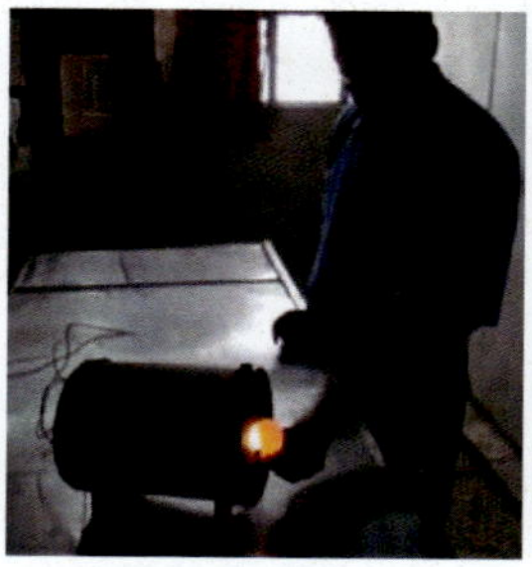

Individual egg candler

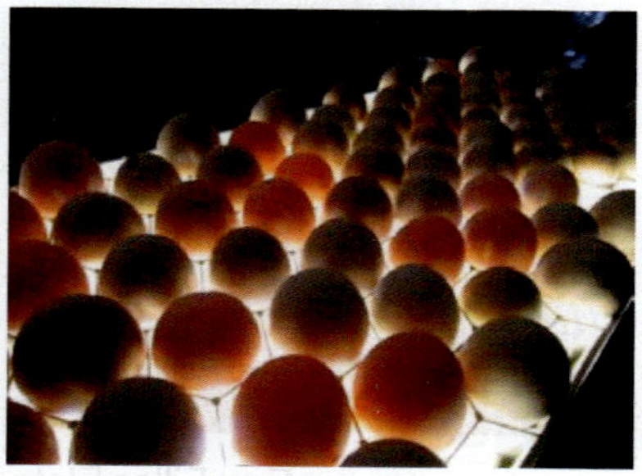

Mass egg Candler

Candling of eggs for grading

Table 1: Egg grades based on weight and quality (AGMARK)

Grade	Weight of one egg (g)	Shell	Air Cell	White	Yolk
A- Extra Large	60 and above	Normal, Clean, unbroken with sound shape	Up to 4 mm in depth, regular or better	Clear, reasonably firm	Fairly well-centred, free from defects, outline clear
A- Large	53-59				
A-Medium	45-52				
A- Small	38-44				
B- Extra Large	60 and above	Slightly abnormal, Clean to moderately stained with sound shape	8 mm in depth, may be free and slightly bubbly	Clear, may be slightly weak	May be slightly off-centred, outline slightly visible
B- Large	53-59				
[illegible]	45-52				
B – Small	38-44				

Packaging of Eggs

Proper packing maintains the quality of the product while helping in handling of the product by the consumer. Packing of eggs depends on the design and materials used as:

1. Basket: Transporting to short distances, eggs can be packed in a simple basket. However, its major disadvantage is the damage to eggs since it does not contain any cushioning material, such as straw. The risk of shell damage can be easily prevented to a greater extent by packing eggs in a basket cushioned with clean and odourless rice husks, wheat chaff or chopped straw.
2. Filler flats: The most common method of packing eggs practised in our country is using filler flats. They may be made up of wood pulp, cardboard or plastic mould. However, plastic egg filler flats are advantageous, as they are reusable and easily washable.

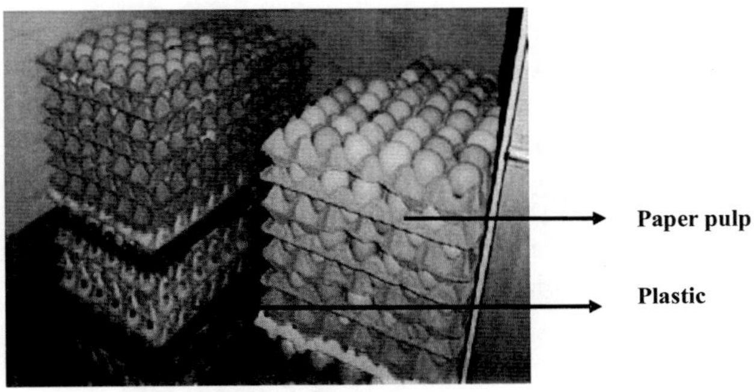

Egg Filler Flats/Trays

One egg filler-flat can accommodate 30 eggs. Usually, filler flats are used for primary packaging and then placed in boxes or cases.

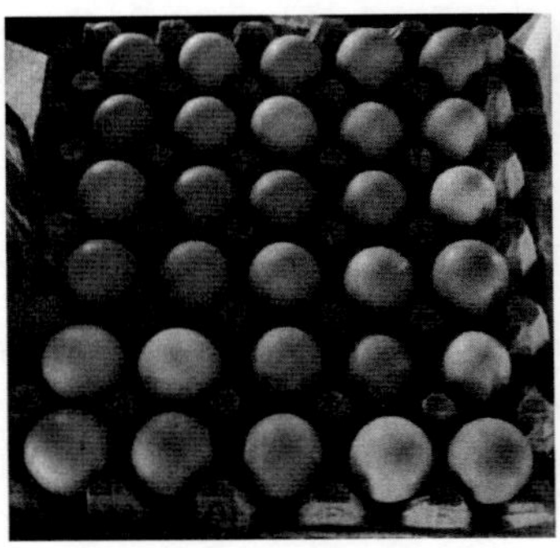

Thirty eggs in one filler flat

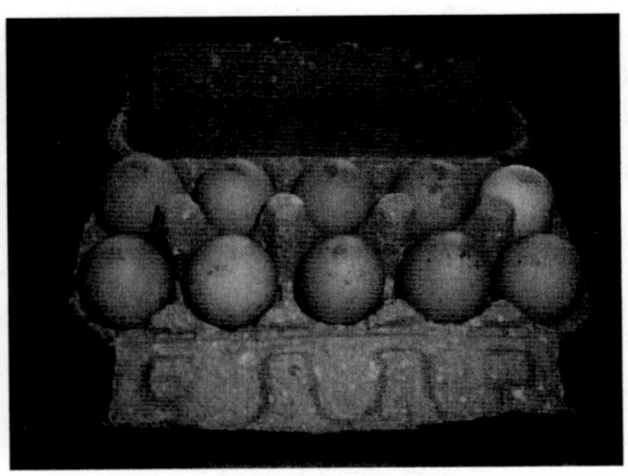

Consumer utility packs

- Cardboard Box: Ten egg filler-flats can be kept in one cardboard box and packed nicely with paper packing, saw dust, dry leaves, etc.
- Paperboard: For retail sale, smaller number of eggs (six to twelve) can be packed in small consumer utility packs made of paperboard or moulded wood pulp so that they are easy to carry. Now-a-days, eggs are packed in small paperboard cases covered with plastic film.

Points to be kept in mind while packing eggs are as follows:

- Only sound, clean and dry containers free from any undesirable smell and insect infestation or fungal contamination should be used.
- The boxes or cartons should be properly labelled "Eggs Handle with Care".
- The basic information like size, weight, quality/grade description of egg, how to store them and the expiry date should be clearly mentioned on the pack.
- The container may be marked with proper instructions, if any, so that the persons may follow these instructions while loading these products on different mode of transportation.

Storage of Eggs

The production of eggs and meat is not throughout the country. About 60% of total poultry production is from the top five poultry egg or meat producing states *viz.* Andhra Pradesh, Haryana, Maharashtra, Punjab and Tamil Nadu. However, these states together accounts to about 30% of total human population. Therefore, the surplus production of perishable products like eggs certainly needs some holding time in the store house for their disposal or consumption. Refrigeration is the best option for storage of eggs for longer periods. The following points should be kept in mind while storing eggs:

·At farm level, after collection, the eggs should be shifted to holding room maintained at a temperature of about 15°C and 70-80% relative humidity for at least 12 hours before shifting to cold store.

- In the cold storage, egg storage area should be cleaned and dried before arrival of eggs.
- The storage room must be free from tainting products/materials and should be cleaned regularly with odourless detergent/ sanitizers.
- The storage area should have adequate power back up.
- The temperature of cold store should be maintained at 4°C and relative humidity between 80-85 per cent.
- In order to maintain the quality of the eggs and to prevent spoilage, it is recommended to maintain proper air circulation in the cold store.
- The eggs placed in cold store should be clean; they must not be washed or made wet.
- Eggs should be stored with the broad end pointing upwards. The quality of shell eggs can be maintained for about 6 months in a cold storage.
- First-in-first-out (FIFO) strategy should be strictly practised so that the oldest eggs are sold first.

Precautions : As eggs have the tendency to absorb odour easily, never store eggs with materials that have distinct odours. Otherwise, the eggs will pick up the odours of apples, fish, onions, potatoes and other food or chemicals with distinct odours.

Transportation of Eggs

Most of the eggs are produced in rural or semi-urban areas, whereas, the consumers are concentrated largely in urban areas. Therefore, the eggs have to be moved from the point of production to the point of consumption. This situation demands use of different modes of transportation. Small quantities can be transported either on head-load, bi/tri-cycles, rickshaws, thelas, tangas, bullock carts (in villages or small towns), etc. However, tractor-trolleys, small vans, trucks, buses, rails, ships and aeroplanes are used for transportation of the major bulk of eggs.

In India, eggs are still transported in open condition and in un-refrigerated vehicles. The entire chain of distribution and physical handling upto the consumer is in open climate exposing eggs to varying temperatures during different seasons. Shelf life of eggs is, therefore, restricted to 11-14 days in summer and 18-20 days in winter. Hence, eggs should be transported in refrigerated vehicles so that their quality does not deteriorate due to high environmental temperatures.

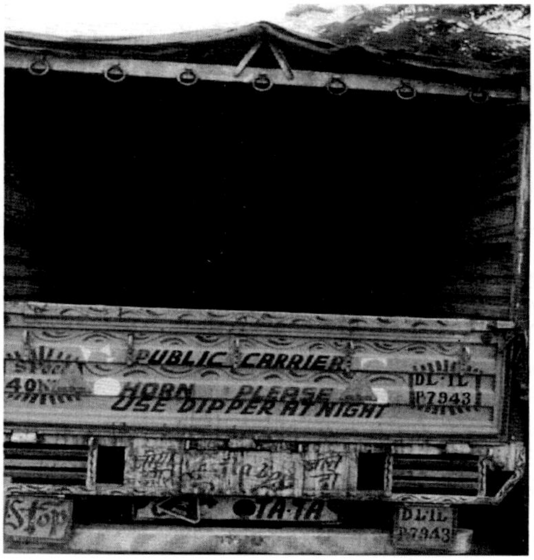

Eggs transported through unrefrigerated truck

It is essential to meet the following three requirements for successful transportation of eggs:

i) Eggs must be well protected against mechanical damage by choosing the right container and packaging material.

ii) Care should be taken at all stages of handling, storage and transport. Since eggs are delicate objects, workers handling eggs should be taught about the importance and need for careful handling of eggs. It is essential to have provision for convenient loading platforms at packing stations, loading depots and railing stations, and handling aids, such as hand trucks and lifts.

iii) Eggs must be protected against exposure to extreme weather conditions, as it may deteriorate the quality as well as may cause contamination.

Do's and Don'ts during transportation of eggs

- While transporting eggs through bicycles, a device, such as a special carrier suspended on springs should be used.

- Clean and disinfect all transport -equipment prior to any egg transport, to avoid contamination.
- While loading the egg boxes or cartons in the vehicle for transportation, utmost care should be taken to lift them with gentle handling.
- Adjust vehicle temperature to that of the storage rooms of all supplying farms.
- Avoid sudden temperature changes during loading and unloading.
- Ensure constant and uniform temperature (1 to 4°C) and humidity (80-85%) during transportation.
- Avoid unnecessary delays.
- Avoid shocks and jolts during loading and transport. Use trucks with good suspension and trolleys with shock absorbing wheels, especially where roads are bad.
- Care is needed to avoid excessive shaking, especially where roads are bad. Egg containers should be stacked tightly and tied down securely to minimize movement. Covers should be used to protect them from the extreme environmental conditions (hot, rain and cold) and adequately support eggs in well-designed trays without sharp edges.
- Do not use sloppy trays and avoid overstacking.
- Always transport eggs with small end down, to avoid loose air cells.
- Use temperature loggers during -transport to record any temperature fluctuations.

❑❑❑

Chapter 17

Processing and Preservation of Poultry Meat

Handling and Transportation of Live Birds

Once the broiler birds attain marketable age (6-8 weeks), they should be properly identified, handled, caught, shifted to crates and transported to the market.

Identifying fit birds

Only fit birds should be marketed. If the sick birds are sold, it may affect the safety of the consumer. Therefore, only healthy and fit birds should be identified and sold. In a flock of broiler birds which has attained marketable age, it is easy to visually identify healthy and unhealthy birds. Healthy birds will be active and alert, move freely and swiftly, consume feed and water normally. Whereas, sick birds will be dull, move away from the group to corners or huddle together, show no or less interest in feed and water, show discharge from eyes/ nose, etc., produce abnormal sounds, showing abnormal postures and behaviour.

Handling of Live Birds

The handling of live birds starts from the production centre (poultry farm) to the point of consumer through the market channels. Handling of birds properly will prevent stress to the birds. Birds selected for slaughter should be procured during the cooler part of the day and transported in crates, preferably plastic crates (Fig.16.10) so that they may not cause any injury or bruises unlike metallic crates. The overcrowding or overloading of birds should be avoided to a maximum extent; otherwise the breast blister is a very common problem and this may downgrade the carcass.

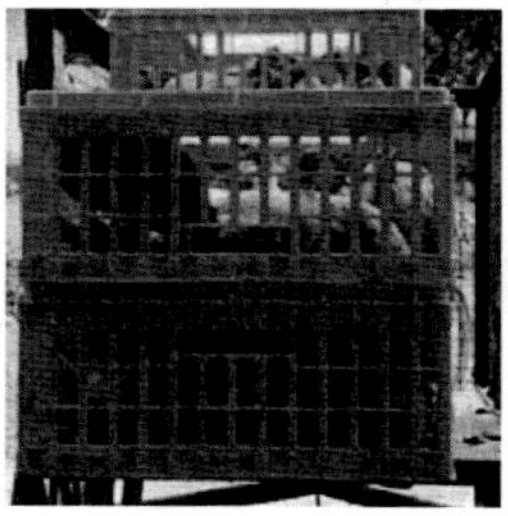

Crate for carrying live birds

Catching and shifting to crates

For catching a bird from a flock in deep litter system, catching mesh and catching hook can be used. During catching, birds are moved to a corner of the shed, and the catching mesh is spread leaving as much space as possible all round so that the birds cannot escape. The birds are then caught using catching hook or by grabbing the legs with fingers. While catching the birds, handle the bird gently to avoid stress and injury. Heavy broiler birds should be held by grabbing the two legs by both the hands. The light birds should be held by one hand by keeping the abdomen of the bird on the palm of one hand and grabbing two legs of bird in between fingers.

Transportation of Live Birds

It is equally important to ensure that the healthy birds reach the consumer or processing plant in sound condition. The quality of birds is affected greatly by the methods employed in transporting them from the farm. Normally, birds are transported through bi/tricycle (Fig.16.11), tractor-trolleys and small vans for shorter distances. However, for distances upto 500 km or 12-15 hours, birds can be transported through road trucks. Whereas, for distances over 500 km, it is advisable to transport birds by rail.

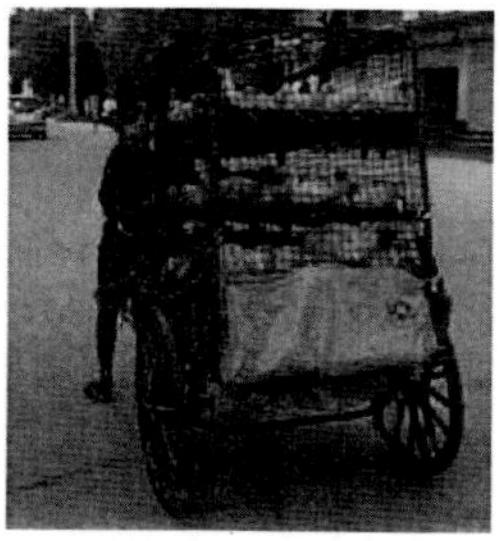

Birds transported by tricycle

The following points need to be kept in mind while transporting live birds:

- Handle the birds gently.
- Do not frighten the birds.
- Birds should be procured and transported during the cooler part of the day.
- Live birds must be transported in a manner that allows for plenty of air ventilation to protect the birds from heat stress. Normally, live birds are transported in metallic (Fig.16.12) or plastic crates (Fig.16.13) constructed so that the birds' legs cannot pass through the bars, but air circulates easily.

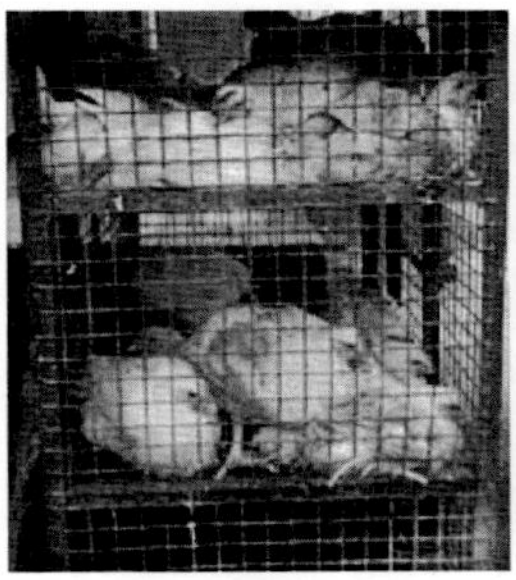

Metallic Crates

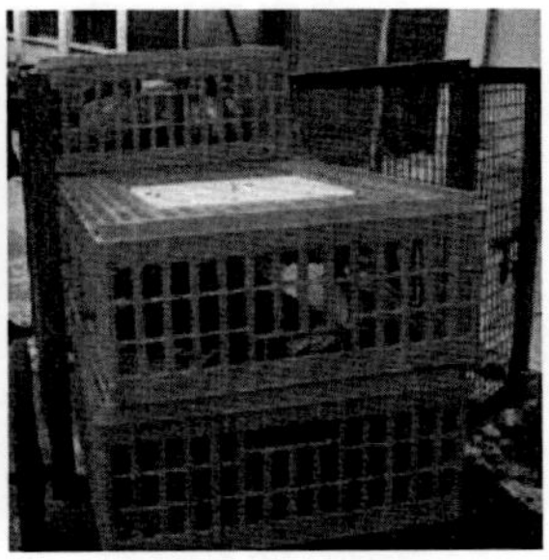

Plastic Crates

- Crates of wire netting on a wood frame are safe, light in weight, and suitable for handling and transport. However, it is preferable to use plastic crates since they do not cause any injury or bruises unlike metallic crates.
- The opening of the crate should be easy to open and close and centrally situated so that all parts of the crate are within reach.
- The dimension of one crate should be 1 m long x 1 m wide x 0.6 m height to accommodate 15-20 adult broilers.
- Considerable death losses, broken wings and legs, and bruises result, if birds are handled roughly or carried in unsuitable or overcrowded containers. Hence, avoid overcrowding or overloading of birds.
- Live birds should be starved for a period of 6 to 8 hours before slaughter. But, sufficient quantity of drinking water should be provided.

Processing of Poultry

The good quality of dressed or ready-to-cook birds can be obtained only from live birds being in prime condition at the time of slaughter. The scientific and hygienic processing of poultry is a must for preserving the quality of meat and to ensure consumer safety and acceptability. The flow sheet for the preparation of ready-to-cook chicken in given below:

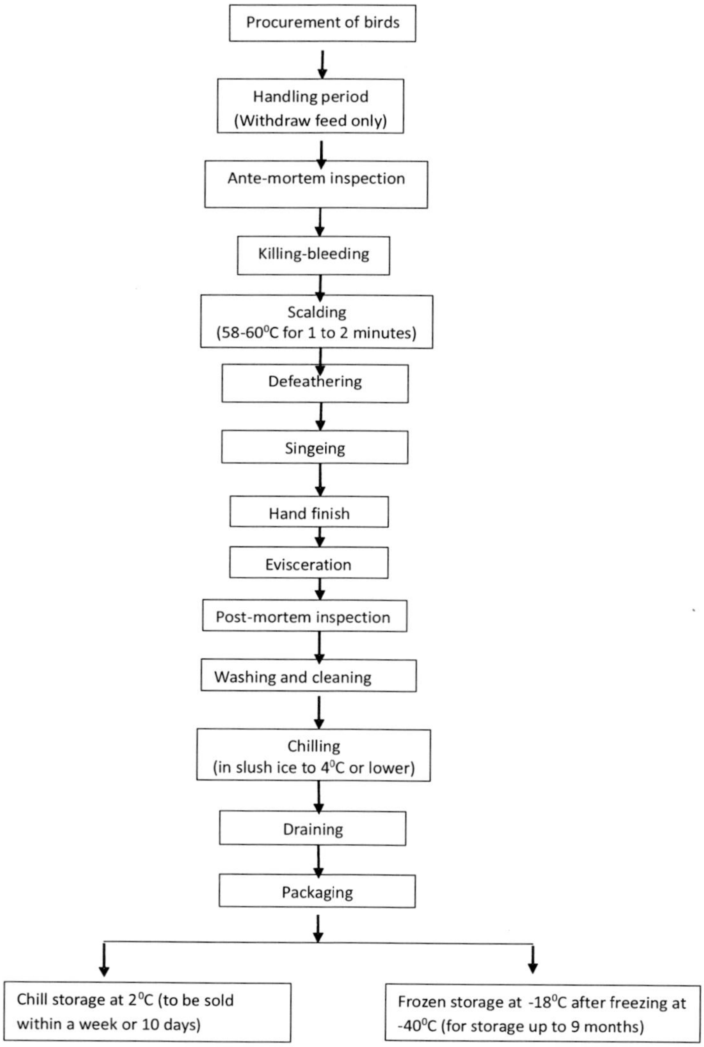

Flow sheet for the preparation of ready-to-cook chicken

Transport

Cages, coops, crates or specially built trucks are used to transport birds from the farm to poultry processing plants. These should be disinfected prior to briging them to the farm to arrest the spread of diseases. Birds should be loaded in dim light to avoid excitement and transported in the cooler hours of the day to prevent excessive loss in weight referred as shrinkage.

Preparing the Birds

Discontinue feed 10-12 hours before the birds are to be killed. Fasting serves to partially empty the digestive tract, thereby reducing the probable risk of rupture of the alimentary tract during evisceration and possible contamination of the carcass with ingesta or faecal matter. Provide plenty of clean and cool drinking water.

Ante-mortem

Birds showing evidence of any disease or any other abnormal condition which may render them unwholesome or unfit for human consumption should be "rejected". The reject, that it is affected by or shows evidence of any disease or condition (including bruises, severe discolouration, severe injuries an emaciation), which may render the bird or any part of it, unfit for human food. The fact that a bird has some condition which causes it to be classified as "rejected" does not necessarily mean that it may be destroyed. Parts or all of the bird might be found, upon evisceration and inspection, to be suitable for human food.

Killing and Bleeding

Generally, poultry is killed by cutting the bird's throat from the outside (outer cut). This is best accomplished by severing the throat and blood vessels (jugular vein and carotid arteries) on both sides of the neck, close to the head using a flat handled sharp edge knife having a small blade. The method of slaughter chosen must also meet the religious requirements of the prospective consumers, such as 'halal' kosher Jhatka, etc. if greater acceptability of processed poultry is to be achieved. Killing is done while the birds are in the bleeding funnels or while suspended from a shackle. It is important to bleed poultry thoroughly after killing.

Electric killing may be beneficial in large plants. It is highly important that the birds are only stunned and not killed. Stumping is done with all electric stunner by applying 90V for half a second.

Scalding

After bleeding and ceasing of all the reflexes the birds are transferred into the scalder, i.e. vessel filled with hot water. The temperature of scald water depends upon the age of the birds. When the temperature is 82-86^{0}C, it is known as hard scalding, when 58-60^{0}C as sub-scalding , when 52-55^{0}C as semi-scalding and when 50-55.5^{0}C soft scalding. The optimum scalding time is 2 minutes.

Scalding at 60^{0}C facilitates the easiest feather plucking but fresh becomes a little tough. This does not occur at lower temperatures (55-57^{0}C). Steam scalding is presently considered to be the best method, as it reduces the total bacterial load on the surface of dressed chicken.

Picking or Plucking or Defeathering

Dry picking or rarely used in commercial organisation. However, when only few birds are done for domestic consumptions, dry picking is still practices.

Wet picking is done either by hand or by mechanical pickers. In hand picking, birds are hung with a cord and block or shackle. Then feathers are removed from different parts in the following order: tail, Wing, sides, legs, back, hips and neck. Mechanical pickers' are used to remove all feathers except the pin feathers: feather plucker machine has two drums with rubber fingers which revolve in opposite directions pulling the feathers on the body in a downward motion.

Pinning

Stubs of feathers are called pin feathers, which must be removed completely to improve the appearance of the carcass. Pin feathers can be removed more easily with a pinning knife (a knife with a shot dull blade). The Pin feathers are held between the knife and the thumb and pulled outwards. Scraping should be avoided, as it produces skin abrasions.

Singeing

Singeing refers to the removal of hair like feathers (filoplumes) by means of a flame. After pinning, the air on the body are removed over a singer or a blow lamp by rotating the carcass over the flame Singeing also causes the destruction or surface microbes and improves appearance and colour of the carcasses.

Washing

The signed carcasses are spray washed before they are put on the evisceration line. This reduces the micro-organisms on carcasses.

Evisceration

The birds should be eviscerated as quickly as possible after slaughter, while they are still warm. Stationery shackle or a table with stainless steel or metal top is used for reasons of sanitation. Large processing plants use an overhead, conveyor line. For marketing whole carcasses, the following evisceration procedure is used:

i) The head and shanks are removed with a sharp knife, meat cleaver or shears.

ii) The skin on the back of the neck is cut from the free end to the base of the neck and the skin is then pulled down to the shoulders.

iii) The gullet, crop and wind pipe are removed by pulling them outwards and cutting off closer to the thoracic cavity.

iv) The neck is disjoined from the body near its origin at the shoulders.

v) The oil gland situated at the base of the tail is removed by cutting under it, deep and backwards towards the tail, to ensure its complete removal.

vi) A transverse cut is made between the keel and the vent, followed by a circular incision around the vent. The viscera are removed through the transverse cut by pulling the gizzard through the opening together with the liver, heart and the gastro-intestinal tract. This removal of internal organs is referred to as drawing. Care should be exercised to avoid rupturing or tearing the intestines, to avoid faecal contamination.

vii) The lungs and kidneys are then removed using the lung Scoop and the kidney retractor.

viii) The carcass is washed inside and out thoroughly with clean water.

ix) The gizzard, liver and heart are removed from the viscera. The gizzard is cut lengthwise and the lining and contents carefully peeled out. Then, the gall bladder is removed from the liver without breaking it. Next to the heart is slit open and emptied of blood. The heart, liver and gizzard are collectively known as giblets.

x) The giblets are washed and wrapped in parchment paper (the neck is also included along the giblets) to be placed in the body cavity.

Trussing

Trussing refers to the fastening or securing of wings and legs to the body with a view to give a more compact and attractive appearance to the carcass. Trussing results in greater case of packing and the processed ready-to-cook carcasses also occupy less space in the freezer, when frozen.

The following steps are required for trussing. The neck skin is drawn as far over the back as possible and the wings are locked over the back to hold the skin in place. The legs of the bird are secured under the fold of skin below the knee. The bird is then ready for chilling.

Cooling or Chilling

Chilling poultry immediately after processing is an important requirement for maintaining top quality. Dressed birds can be chilled in cold water, crushed ice, slush ice, solid carbon dioxide to cool down the carcass to an internal temperature of 2.2-4.4^{0}C in about 45 minutes. The chilled birds are then kept for sometime on draining rack to remove excess water.

Wrapping or Packing

Wrapping of poultry meat in a suitable packing affords a certain amount of protection to the contents during storage distribution and sales. Selection of packaging material depends on the criteria of its physical strength, permeability to water vapour and other gases, transparency, cold resistance and heat sealing property. Some of the very commonly used flexible packing materials are polythylenefilm, shrinkable polyethylene, polyethylene, polyvinylidine, polystyrene and cellophane, chilled and drained birds are vacuum packed in one of these packaging materials depending upon the availability.

Physical appearance of birds sometimes gives false impression. This necessitates the examination of carcass after slaughter. This is called post-mortem inspection. Birds showing any clinical evidence of disease on post-mortem should be condemned.

Processing losses and yields

The proportion of dresses, carcass weight to live body weight is often used as a measure of meat production. Percentage of edible carcass remaining after dressing and evisceration is of great value to producers, processors and consumers. Weightloss represented by, inedible parts of chicken may well form the basis for pricing system in the marketing of processed poultry.

i) Shrinkage-May be defined as loss of weight.

ii) Fasting shrinkage-Is the weightloss resulting from fasting birds immediately before slaughter.

iii) Procurement shrink-Is weightloss due to transportation of live birds from the farm to the slaughter unit.

iv) Dressing losses-Those represented by loss of weight due to removal of blood and leathers. Dressing losses vary from 5-10% live weight.

v) Evisceration shrink-is weightloss resulting from the removal of head, feet (including shanks) and viscera.

vi) Dressing and drawing losses-Consist of losses due to blood, feathers, head, feet and viscera. Dressing and drawing losses are known to vary with breed, age, condition of fleshing, sex, etc. on an average, dressing and drawing losses may vary between 25 to 35% of the live weight.

Poultry meat quality

The quality characteristic of poultry meat refers to appearance, texture, juiciness, flavour, nutritive value, wholesomeness, meat to bone ratio, etc. of the palatability factors, texture is more important which is influenced by the genetic make-up of birds, sex, age, muscular activity, nutrition, management treatments prior to slaughter, such as physical stress during catching and transport, pre-slaughter factors like methods of killing, bleeding, scalding, plucking, chilling and ageing.

The factors affecting quality of meat are given below:

Tearing and disfigurement

Tearing occurs due to overcrowding either during transportation or processing of birds or due to defective rubber fingers of 'the feather plucker machine. Such carcasses become susceptible to bacterial contamination or decomposition.

Poor bleeding

Poorly bled carcasses have poor keeping quality and unattractive appearance. Poor bleeding may be due to improper slaughter or too little time allowed for bleeding.

Over-scalding

Over-scald carcasses have a partially cooked superficial skin and are more susceptible to bacterial growth and decomposition.

Freezer burn

When frozen poultry is stored for a period of time under severely fluctuating temperatures, evaporation of moisture from the skin of the carcass may be so great that light coloured, pockmarks appear on the skin. Such a condition is called freezer burn and it is an outstanding visual defect of refrigerated poultry.

Since most of the moisture in frozen products is in a solid state, little, if any moisture moves to the surface to replace that lost by surface evaporation. This results in the uneven dehydration of the skin around the feather follicles, giving rise to this defect. It has been reported that severely freezer-burned muscle tissue contains only 50-55% moisture, whereas normal tissue contains about 72%. Dried out meat becomes tough and hard to cook, accompanied by loss of flavour, tenderness and juiciness. Apart from these, carcasses showing freezer burn condition have a poor eye-appeal and consequently reduce the sale value of such poultry.

Packing poultry in a moisture-proof wrapper and quick freezing are the best ways to reduce freezer burns.

Off flavour

It may be caused by rancidity, contamination decomposition and absorption of extraneous odours either at the time of processing storage.

Grading, packaging, storage and transport

The processed ready-to-cook chicken is graded for confirmation, degree of fleshing and other quality attributes. The BIS standards (table: 16.1) or dressed chicken should be followed for this purposes. They are packed individually either in polyethylene bags of medium density or vacuum-packaged in heat shrinkable film-bags. Carcasses can be stored for 7-10 days at -2 ^{0}C, but for longer storage (5-8 months) they are deep frozen at (minus 40^{0}C) and stored at -17 to -18^{0}C.

For short distance transport insulated containers of suitable thermal efficiency provided with adequate refrigeration can be used. Refrigerated vehicles are used for long distance transport. Chickens are marketed as live and ready-to-cook forms. Now-a-days, cut up parts of processed chicken viz., breast, thigh, drum stick (legs) wings, back and giblet are also being sold.

Table 1: Bureau of Indian standards for dressed chicken

Grade 1	Grade 2
a) Confirmation	***a) Confirmation***
Free of deformities that detract from its appearance or that affect the normal distribution of flesh. Slight deformities, such as slightly curved or dented breast bones and slightly curved backs may be present.	Slight abnormalities, such as dented: curved or cooked breast, crooked back, or mis-shapen legs or wings, which do not materially affect the distribution of flesh or the appearance of the carcass or part.
b) Fleshing	***b) Fleshing***
The breast is moderately long and deep, and has sufficient flesh to give it a rounded appearance with the flesh carrying well upto the crest of the breast bone along at its entire	The breast has a substantial covering of flesh with the flesh carrying upto the crest of the breast bone sufficiently to prevent a thin appearance.

c) Fat covering	*c) Fat covering*
The fat is well distributed so that there is a noticeable amountof fat in the skin in the areas between the heavy feather tracts.	The fat under the sin is sufficient to prevent a distinct appearance of the flesh through the skin, especially-on the breast and legs.
d) Defeathering	*d) Defeathering*
Free of pill feathers, diminutive feathers, and hair which are visible to the inspector or grader.	Not more than an occasional protruding pin feather or diminutive feathers shall be in evidence under a careful examination.
e) Cuts and tears	*e) Cuts and tears*
Free of cuts and tears on the breast.	The carcass may have very few cuts and tears.
f) Discolouration	*f) Discolouration*
Free from discolouration dale to bruising free of clots; flesh bruises and discolouration of the skin, such as 'blue black' are not permitted on the breast or legs of the carcass or on these individual parts and only lightly shaded discolorations are permitted elsewhere.	Discoloration dale to bruising; freed of clots; moderate areas of discolouration due to bruises in the skin or flesh and moderately shaded discoloration of the skin, such as 'blue black' are permitted.
g) Freezer burn	*g) Freezer burn*
May have ail occasional pock marks due to drying of the inner layer of skin (provided that none exceed the area of a circle 0.5cm in diameter on Chickens.	May have a few pock marks due to drying of the inner layer of skin (derma), provided that no single area exceeds that of a circle 1.5 cm in diameter.

Preservation of poultry meat

The primary objective of poultry meat preservation is to inhabit microbial spoilage and arrest physio-chemical processes, which bring about deterioration in quality. Some of the methods followed for preservation of poultry meat are described below:

Refrigeration

Crushed ice of mechanical refrigeration is generally used for chilling or cool storage of meat. Poultry meat can be stored at 1-4^{0}C (35-40^{0}F) with relative humidity of 80-85 per cent for about a week. The effectiveness of refrigeration storage can be increased by modifying the storage atmosphere by introducing 10-12 per cent carbon dioxide in the atmosphere.

Freezing

Poultry meat can be frozen in air or liquid or refrigerated plates. Only chilled carcasses should be frozen. Slow freezing with still air, the method generally utilised is some freezer or small freezing operation, results in a product of poor quality. On quick freezing methods, air blast system is widely used in commercial freezing of poultry meat. The pre-packaged carcasses are blast frozen at -30 to -40°C with an air velocity of 1300-1500 rpm in about 2 to 3 hours and stored unaltered through intracellular ice formation. Quick frozen broilers could be stored at -20°C for 12, 15 and 1.8 months with excellent, good and satisfactory quality respectively.

Curing and smoking

These are closely inter-related and often practiced together. Curing is the process of salting meat along with one or more of the glutamates, ascorbic acid, acetic acid and phosphates. The curing room temperature is maintained at 31°C Chicken can be dry or wet cured. In dry curing, the curing mixture is rubbed thoroughly on the surface of carcasses and aged. In wet or pickle curing, the curing solution is either injected in small quality at several places into the meat or the carcasses are immersed in a curing solution.

The smoking process imparts a characteristic flavour and stable colour to the cured product and aids in preservation by the combined action of heat and smoke components, such as phenols, aldehydes, organic acids, lower alcohols and carbonyl compounds.

Cured chicken could be stored for 4 and 14 days at ambient (26°C) and refrigeration (4-5°C) temperatures respectively, and cured and smoked chicken for 14 and 30 days under the corresponding storage conditions.

Dehydration

Conventional hot air, drum, spray and freeze drying are the methods used in the dehydration of poultry meat. Generally cooked meat is dehydrated. Drying of raw meat results in surface hardening, poor dehydration and acceptability. Cooked chicken chunks or ground chicken meat spread in these layers on pans or trays are dried in a rotary air drier with controlled temperature and air flow to a moisture content of 5%. Spray drying of finely ground cooked meat results in a product suitable for preparation of chicken soup.

Canning

It is heat processing of meat in sealed containers.

Use of antibiotics

Antibiotics can be used for the preservation of raw meat but not in processed products. The antibiotics used not impart off-colour off-flavour, and should be non-toxic, stable, soluble and effective at the pH of meat. A low level of chlortetracycline or oxytetracycline is suitable for meat preservation at chilling temperature.

The problem associated with antibiotics preservation are the development of resistant strains of bacteria, changes in intestinal flora and sensitization to antibiotics. However, there is remote possibility of such effect since they are destroyed during cooking, leaving no harmful end products.

Radiation preservation

The radiant energy is used to destroy the micro-organisms and inactivate enzymes without any rise in the temperature of foods. It is also known as cold sterilisation. This method is used as a supplement to the other methods, such as refrigeration, freezing and canning. This method is expensive.

Tenderization

The tough meat of culled and spent birds (birds which have completed egg production) is made tender by the use of various proteolytic enzymes either alone or in combination.

❑❑❑

Chapter **18**

Record Keeping

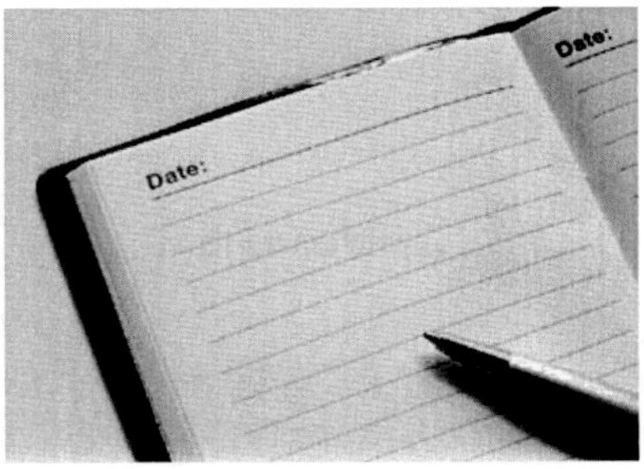

Farm business records keeping refer to documentation of events, business or news that occurs on the farm, and it is a crucial step in the success of every farming business. Farm records keeping provides the farmer with a tool to help in farm planning, farm management decision making, and projection of future profitability of the enterprise, with an aim of maximizing farm profit. Records are important to the financial health of a business or operation. Efficient and profitable poultry operations are not guaranteed by good record keeping, but success is unlikely without them. Records are essential tools for management to maintain a successful flock. Record keeping involves keeping, filing, maintaining, and categorizing inventory, financial and production information for your flock. This can be accomplished by hand recording or by using computer software.

A good record provides data to assess financial ability of business operation analysis, assists in obtaining loans, measure profitability, file income tax return and overall decision- making process.

Purposes of Records

1. Measure profit and access the financial ability of the business/ operation.
2. Provides data for business/operation analysis.
3. Assists in obtaining loans.
4. Measure the profitability of individual operation.
5. Assist in analysis of new investments.
6. Help prepare income tax returns.

Two types of records are maintained on the farm:

i) Account records for accountancy and

ii) Technical records to evaluate performance of birds.

Accountancy records are : (i) Balance sheet (ii) Receipts (iii) Expenses. They are summarized on monthly or yearly basis to show the financial status of the farm.

Technical records are : (i) Feed record (ii) Grower flock record (iii) Layer flock record (iv) Incubation record (v) Vaccination record (vi) yearly assessment record.

Traditionally, poultry farmers maintain have kept records by hand which is still useful for many farmers. Yet, the use of computers and computer software has expanded on farms in recent years because of better record accuracy. The farm manager decides on the system that best fits his/her situation.

Hand-Recording System

- Low initial out-of-pocket expense
- Easy to start
- Requires only pencil & paper

Computer Recording System

- More accurate & faster
- Tax deductible as an expense
- Much easier to create analysis

Following daily records should be monitored in a poultry farm:

- Feed consumption
- Water consumption
- Maximum and minimum temperature
- Mortality and laboratory diagnostic reports
- Medication
- Vaccination

- Feed, gas, litter deliveries, etc.
- Body weight records
- Record on a flock basis
- Electricity usage
- Gas/oil usage
- Stocking density

Record maintenance is a crucial activity in any business. It will serve as important source for monitoring and evaluation. A business can be efficiently managed, only if proper recording of data is carried out periodically. The records maintained are primarily a documentation of accountability and secondarily a *data system* for management. They should be reliable and relevant. This relevant information, when recorded, should be made available at any time. Records should be simple, easy to understand, without repetition; but must provide all the needed information. The records should be able to clearly state, where and how the enterprise stands. The history of the record will provide the entrepreneur, a clear picture of all mistakes made in the past and to be avoided in future. The records are necessary to study the production performance, and check whether it meets the prescribed standards. Records should provide information for future planning, changes and expansions, if any.

In general, farm records can be broadly classified under two categories:

- Production/ Technical records
- Financial records

The nature of the records varies, based on the type and volume of the enterprise.

Irrespective of the type and size of enterprises, the basic records to be maintained are as follows:

Attendance and daily wage register

This deals with the number of persons employed daily and wages dispersed to them; including the stamped acquaintance.

Building Registers

- This deals with the various farm buildings and other civil works like well, fencing, roads, etc.
- In this register one has to maintain the petty repairs and expenditure incurred for their maintenance.
- Moreover, the annual depreciation on buildings should also be worked out every year.
- After deducting the annual depreciation, the actual worth of the buildings should be brought forward for various accounting purposes.

Equipment Register

- This includes various farm equipment machineries like feed mill, vehicles, cages, incubators, feeders, waterers, etc.
- The date, source, number and cost of purchase of equipment must be recorded.
- The repairs carried out along with the details of repairs also must be indicated.
- The annual depreciation should be calculated for equipment and the actual post-depreciation value for equipment must be brought forward for the next year.

Feed and feed ingredient register

Feed is the major item of expenditure in poultry production. Hence, much care should be exercised in maintaining this register. Few pages must be allotted for each feed ingredient of the feed.

For each of these items, the opening balance, receipts, issues, storage loss, manufacturing cost and the closing balance has to be maintained. In the remarks column, the source of purchase, invoice number and date and cost per unit must be indicated. Since the feed ingredient prices vary frequently, the actual ingredient cost for each batch of feed mixed must be taken into account, for accurate calculation.

Feed additives and medicines register

This register keeps track of the various feed additives, medicines, vaccines, disinfectants, chemicals purchased and utilized.

The opening balance, receipts, issues, closing balance and a remarks column must be maintained for each item. In the remarks column, the invoice number, date, cost and source of each purchase have to be indicated.

Layer farm register

For each batch, the production performance register has to be maintained from day one to disposal; with the following columns:

Date, age in days, opening balance of birds, mortality, feed issued, feed/ bird/ day, eggs produced, % Hen-day egg production, Feed/ egg and remarks. The remarks column should deal with date of vaccinations, debeaking, medication, post-mortem report, if any, sale of culled birds and any other relevant information. A separate book has to be maintained for each batch from day one to disposal, so that batch wise economics can be calculated.

Broiler farm records

For broiler farms, batch wise performance sheet has to be maintained, with the following columns. Before the regular columns, the batch number, source of chicks, number of paid and free chicks received, date of hatch, cost per chick and strain, have to be recorded.

The regular data to be recorded are date, age in days, opening balance of birds, mortality, total feed issued and remarks. In the remarks column, the medication and vaccination details, cause of death may be indicated. These regular columns should continue upto 56 days; but recording should be done until the date of sale.

Below these regular columns the following particulars like total live body weight of birds sold, number of birds sold, per cent mortality, total feed consumed, feed conversion ratio, cost of feed, sale price of broilers sold, cost of chicks and miscellaneous cost (electricity, labour, medicine, vaccination, fuel, etc.) have to be recorded.

Based on the above data, the actual cost of production/ kg live weight and the profit/ loss incurred for that batch has to be calculated.

It is good practice for all processes in a broiler operation to have standard operation protocol (SOP). These should include documentation of established procedures, records, record analysis and monitoring system.

Table 1: Records Required in Broiler Production

Event	Records	Comments
Chick placement	Number of day –olds Flock of origin and age Date and time of arrival Chick quality Crop fill	Live weight, uniformity, number of dead on arrival Check crop fill percentage
Mortality	Daily Weekly Cumulative	Record by sex if possible Record culls with reasons Post-mortem records of excess mortality Scoring of coccidial lesions will indicate level of coccidial challenge Record actual numbers and percentages Particular importance should be given to 7-day mortality
Medication	Date Amount Batch number	As per veterinary instructions
Vaccination	Date of vaccination Vaccine type Batch number	Any unexpected vaccine reaction should be recorded.
Live weight	Weekly average live weight Weekly uniformity	More frequent measurement is required when predicting weight
Feed	Date of purchase Quantity Feed type Feed form Date of starting feed withdrawal	Accurate measurement of feed consumed to measure FCR and to determine cost effectivenss of broiler operation. Check feed quality
Water	Daily consumption Water to feed ratio Water quality Level of chlorination	Plot daily consumption graph Sudden fluctuation in water consumption is an early indication of a problem Mineral and/or bacteriological when bore wells or open water reservoir is used
Environment	Temperature Floor as well as litter Daily minimum/ maximum During brooding Relative humidity Air quality Litter quality	Multiple locations should be monitored Automatic systems should be cross checked manually Ideally record dust, NH3
Depletion	Number of birds removed Time and date of removal	
Information from processing plant	Carcass quality Health inspection Carcass composition Type and % condemnation	

Cleaning out	Total bacterial count	After disinfection, salmonella, staphylococcus or E.coli may be monitored
House inspection	Record time of daily checks Make note of any bird observations	Behaviour and environmental conditions
Lighting programme	Dark and light periods Time on and time off	Intermittent or not
Visitors	Who Why Date and reason of visit Previous farm visit	Should be completed for every visitor

Breeder farm records

The records will be similar to that of the layer farm. However, one more column, namely the number of hatching eggs produced daily has to be included in the batch wise performance and egg out turn register.

Hatchery records

The hatchery should maintain a register similar to that of egg out turn register but with some modified columns as follows:

Date, opening balance, receipts, settings, discards and sales, chicks produced, chicks sold, chicks discarded, free chicks and remarks.

Batch wise hatchery sheet

This may be maintained, to provide the following information:

Serial setting number, number of eggs set, type of eggs, strain, source of eggs, number of eggs discarded, number of eggs transferred to hatcher, number of good chicks hatched, number of weak chicks, number of pullet chicks (in case of egg-type only), number of male chicks and mode of disposal, per cent total hatchability and per cent fertility.

Chick out turn and disposal register

This register consists of strain wise chick out turn and disposal particulars, consisting of date, opening balance of chicks, chicks hatched, chicks sold, chicks used for own purpose, chicks discarded, chicks given as free margin, closing balance, price per chick and remarks.

The remarks column should have the Marek's disease vaccination and other particulars.

Feed mill record

The feed mill registers will be similar to the general registers discussed above but with more details about individual feed ingredients. Instead of maintaining few pages for each ingredient and feed in the same register, a separate register has to be maintained for each ingredient and feed. An extra column showing the feed ingredient shortage due to storage, grinding and mixing loss has to be indicated at the expiry of each batch or lot received or mixed. Moreover, the remarks column must indicate the source of purchase, bill number, unit price and mode of payment, in case of feeding ingredient. In case of different feeds prepared – to whom sold, quality, rate per unit, invoice number and mode of receipt should be indicated.

Economic Indices for a Broiler Farm

The farmer will be interested in knowing at what position his farm stands on economic grounds and the efficiency of his farm operates. The following methods and formulae may be used as tools to measure the performance of the birds:

1. Feed Conversion ratio

This is the most important and commonly sued efficiency measure in a broiler farm. It is calculated by using the formula:

$$FCR = \frac{\text{Total feed consumed in kg}}{\text{Total body weight in kg}}$$

A value of less than 2.00 at 6 weeks of age is preferable. Lower the value better will be the efficiency.

2. Performance Index (P.I)

It is the ratio of live weight in Ibs and feed conversion ratio multiplied by 100

$$P.I = \frac{\text{Live Weight in Ibs}}{\text{Feed Conversion ratio}} \times 100$$

Higher the value better will be the index. A value of 200 and above is desirable.

3. Broiler Performance Efficiency Factor (BPEF)

It is the ratio of live weight in kg to the feed conversion efficiency multiplied by 100

$$\text{BPEF} = \frac{\text{Live weight in kg}}{\text{Feed Conversion ratio}} \times 100$$

Higher the value better will be the index. A value of 100 and above is desirable.

4. Construction Coefficient (CC)

It is the ratio of total constructed area to the total farm land area multiplied by 100

$$\text{CC} = \frac{\text{Total constructed area}}{\text{Total farmland area}} \times 100$$

Construction coefficient should be 25 to 35 for an ideal farm. A higher value indicates congestion, overcrowding, poor ventilation and more diseases. Lower value is suggestive of poor utilization of land which means higher investment on land per bird.

5. Gross Margin per Unit Floor Area

Gross margin per unit floor area depends upon the stocking density, growth rate, mortality and the market prices for the outputs.

$$\text{Gross Margin/m2} = \frac{\text{Total receipts/year}}{\text{Total floor area (m2)}}$$

Higher the value, better will be the efficiency

6. Point Spread (PS)

PS= Live weight in Lbs-Feed conversion ratio x100

A value of 200 or more is considered to be more economical. If the live weight is expressed in Kg, the PS will be near to zero or even a negative value. Hence, it is not advised to calculate PS with metric units.

7. Benefit-Cost ratio (BCR)

It is the ratio between total gross receipts and the total expenditure incurred by the farm.

A value of one BCR indicates no profit or loss.

More than one indicates profits

Less than one indicates loss to farm

Value of 1.20 and above are desirable.

8. Broiler Feed Price ratio (BFPR)

$$\text{BFPR} = \frac{\text{Total value of meat or live chicken produced}}{\text{Total value of feed}}$$

Higher body weight gain, lower mortality, better feed efficiency, lower feed cost and higher selling price results in a favourable BFPR value. A value of more than 2 is desirable.

9. Broiler Performance Efficiency Index (BPEI)

$$\text{BPEI} = \frac{\text{Total sealable live weight (kg)}}{\text{No of chicks purchased x Feed efficiency}}$$

A BPEI value of 100 or higher is desirable

10. Formula for calculating cost of production/kg Live Broiler

Chick cost=0.55 x cost of one day old chick = A

Feed cost=Feed efficiency x cost/kg of feed = B

Miscellaneous expenditure=Add 12% A+B =C

Therefore, production cost/kg live broiler = A+B+C

11. Formula for calculating cost of production/Broiler

Chick cost=1.05 x cost of day old chick=A

Feed cost=Live weight (kg) x Feed x cost/kg of feed efficiency=B

Miscellaneous expenditure=

Add 12% of A+B=C

Therefore, production cost/kg Broiler= A+B+C

12. Formula for calculating cost of production/kg ready to cook broiler

$$\text{Cost of one kg RTC} = \frac{1+\text{ cost of one live chicken}}{\text{Live weight (Kg) x 0.73}}$$

13. Broiler Farm Economy index (BFEI)

$$\text{BFEI} = \frac{\text{Average live weight (kg) x (percent Liveability}}{\text{Feed Efficiency x Growth period (days)}}$$

A BFEI value of 2 and above indicates better management value of less than 1.3 indicates poor performance.

Economic Indices for a Layer Farm

1. Feed efficiency (FE) / Kg egg mass

- It is the ratio between the feed consumed and the egg mass in Kg.
- This takes into consideration the feed intake, egg weight and egg production.
- A value of 2.2 or less is advantageous to the farm.

$$\text{FE/kg egg mass} = \frac{\text{Kg. of feed consumed}}{\text{Kg. of egg produced}}$$

2. Feed Efficiency (FE) / dozen eggs

- It is the feed consumed per dozen eggs.
- It is the most commonly used index in layers.
- The value should be 1.5 or less in a well maintained farm.

$$\text{FE/dozen eggs} = \frac{\text{Kg. of feed consumed for every}}{\text{12 eggs produced}}$$

3. Hen Day Egg Production (HDEP)

- It is the percentage of eggs produced by the survivor population.
- It can be expressed both in number and percentage.

- A farm or flock average of 85% or 310 eggs per year or above are desirable.

$$H.D.E.P/Day = \frac{\text{No. of eggs produced}}{\text{Total no. of live hens on that day}} \times 100$$

$$H.D.E.P/Period = \frac{\text{Total number of eggs produed during a period}}{\text{Total number of hen days during that period}} \times 100$$

(sum of opening balance of live hens one ach day)

4. Hen Housed Egg Production (HHEP)

- It is the egg production, based on the initial number of hens housed in the flock.
- It can be expressed both in number and percentage. H.H.E.P.
- Values of 295 or 80% or higher are desirable.

$$H.H.E.P/Day = \frac{\text{No. of eggs produced on a given day}}{\text{Total number of hens hosed at the beginning}} \times 100$$

$$H.H.E.P/Period = \frac{\text{Average daily number of eggs produced/day}}{\text{No. of hens housed initially}} \times 100$$

5. Net Feed Efficiency index

$$NFEI = \frac{\text{Mean egg mass (g) + Mean body weight}}{\text{Average Feed consumption x 100}}$$

NFEI value of 45 and above is desirable

6. Performance Efficiency index

This is based on the data on egg weight, body weight, egg production and feed consumption

$$PEI = \frac{30(EW)^{2P}}{BWxF}$$

EW=Average egg weight (g)

BW=Average body weight (g)

P= Percentage hen-day egg production

F=Average Feed consumed/day in g

7. Egg: Feed Price Ratio

$$EFPR = \frac{\text{Total value of eggs produced}}{\text{Total value of feed consumed}}$$

8. Egg Mass/Hen housed

Kilograms of eggs produced/hen housed

9. Formula for calculating Production cost of egg

Production cost of one egg =

$$\frac{\text{Total feed consumption in the laying year x feed cost/kg} + \text{Total of other inputs (25\% of feed cost)}}{\text{Total no of eggs produced}}$$

❑❑❑

Chapter 19

Entrepreneurship and Marketing

During the current years, poultry production has taken the shape of Industry due to high demand and good returns. Now-a-days chicken meat and eggs are food items while few years ago, it was considered as only livestock product. Commercial poultry production is a highly competitive business that involves substantial investment of capital and a considerable element of risk. The demand for high quality eggs and broilers is growing along with the increase in population. Before entering into poultry farming, its benefits and limitations should be borne in mind. Location of the farm, genetic stock, feed quality, size of operation, layout efficiency, mortality rate among the flock and price of the produce (egg and meat) are the major factors affecting profitability in a poultry farm.

Economics and Finance for Poultry Farming

Indian Poultry Industry has three major segments:

- Broilers
- Layers
- Backyard poultry

Broiler Industry

Poultry meat is an important source of high quality proteins, minerals and vitamins for balanced human diet. Specially developed varieties of chicken (broilers) are now available with the traits of quick growth and high feed conversion efficiency. Depending on the farm size, broiler farming can be a main source of family income or can provide subsidiary income and gainful employment to farmers throughout the year. The commercial broiler chicks are ready in less than 40 days. Feed (65%) and chicks (25%) account for 90% of the broiler inputs and the consolidation started in the production. There is a wide gap between the economics of the smaller units purchasing feed & chicks and the ones using their own feed & chicks. Big companies with larger investments came in and the smaller units compromised on growing the broilers for the company on the contract basis, restricting themselves to the 10% of the production cost. This synergy in the form of "Contract Farming" is an excellent development that took place in India. Farmers with small land-holding find growing broilers on "All-in-All-out" basis for a company, in a poultry house built on the land is giving better and assured returns compared to agriculture, which is more nature-dependent and uncertain.

The advantages of broiler farming are:

- Initial investment is a little lower than layer farming.
- Rearing period is 5-6 weeks only.
- More number of flocks can be taken in the same shed.
- Broilers have high feed conversion efficiency i.e. the amount of feed required for unit body weight gain is lower in comparison to other livestock.
- Faster return from the investment.
- Demand for poultry meat is more compared to sheep/goat meat.

There is a growing trend of integration in broiler farming. In the early nineties, contract farming for broilers was introduced and in 1995 it spread all over Tamil Nadu. Between 1995 and 2000, it spread to Karnataka. It gathered momentum and spread its wings to Maharashtra, Andhra Pradesh in the years 2001 & 2002 and after that, it gained inroads into West Bengal and Gujarat. The spread is due to built in strengths in integration system. Integrators will take care of all aspects of production, right from raising of grandparent and parent flocks, production of day old chicks for rearing, manufacturing and supply of concentrate feed, providing veterinary services and wholesale marketing of birds. Under contract farming, poultry farmers invest only for poultry sheds / equipment on their existing land. The Integrator supplies chicks, feed, medicines, provides technical guidance and takes entire production after 5-6 weeks.

The contract farmers are paid growing charges as per agreed rates. This has eliminated the middlemen. Farmer is benefiting from the lesser investment and production cost and also higher productivity, which are achieved as a result of integration. However, the farmer may be at a disadvantage, if the number of batches supplied in the year by the integrator is less.

The feed & chicken prices go up. The chicken prices move very slowly. The gap is being met with efficiency in production.

Small scale poultry (broiler) farm: In some parts of country, there are some entrepreneurial models which promote poultry by small farmers. Costing for a small batch of 500/1000 birds. They support in building a conventional shed at cost around Rs.10,000. Then they provide all inputs like (chicks, feed and support) one cycle in advance. If you make agreement with some company like Suguna, etc. they will give 5 batches per year and 2.5 rupees per KG (Weight of Bird). In average for 40 days, the hen weigh about 2 KG. i.e. 5000 birds x 2 Kg/bird x 2.5 rupee=25000/batch +5000 manure = 30000 Expenditure per batch is around 10,000 rupees (includes labour) Total profit per batch is Rs. 20,000/- If you are doing by own than expenditure for 5000 birds is around 5 lac per batch and you can earn as per market price (that is vary, today price is 70) As per present rate, you can earn around 3 to 4 lakhs per batch.

But there are two different things:

1. Poultry farming at smaller scale, where investments are less, profits are less and management is easy.

Commercial poultry faraming, where investment are huge and returns and risks are too very huge and the management is very extensive.

Economics of Broiler Farming

(10,000 Broilers per cycle)

A- CAPITAL COST

S.No.	Capital Cost (for 08 years)	Rate	Total
1.	At least 1 acre of the land for 8 year (Ideally it should be in some distant rural areas)	Rs. 10,000/- per acre per year	Rs.80,000/-
2.	Fencing of the 1 acre land	Rs. 25,000/-	Rs. 25,000/-
3.	Construction of the Brooder cum grower house one sq. ft. per bird for 10,000 birds	Rs. 200/- per sq ft	Rs. 20,00,000/-
4.	Jetpump / Borewell with submersible pump	Rs. 45,000/- + Rs. 15,000/-	Rs. 60,000/-
5.	Water Pipelines in the shed & outside	Rs. 50,000/-	Rs. 50,000/-
6.	Water storage tank installed above the building	Rs. 40,000/-	Rs. 40,000/-
7.	Feeder/ Waterer / Brooder for ten thousand birds	Rs. 10/- per bird	Rs. 1,00,000/-
8.	Electrification	Rs. 50,000/-	Rs. 50,000/-
9.	Feed/ Medicine Store 200 sq ft	Rs. 200/- per sq ft	Rs. 40,000/-
10.	Office cum product selling room 10×12 feet	Rs. 200/- per sq ft	Rs. 24,000/-
11.	Power back up (Inverter & Generator)	Rs. 20,000/- + Rs. 80,000/-	Rs. 1,00,000/-
12.	Refrigerator	Rs. 11,000/-	Rs. 11,000/-
13.	Miscellaneous Expenditure	Rs. 50,000/-	Rs. 50,000/-
		Total Capital Cost	**Rs. 26,30,000/-**

B- EXPENDITURE

S.No.	Items	Duration							
		1st Year	2nd Year	3rd Year	4th Year	5th Year	6th Year	7th Year	8th Year
1.	Cost of day old chick @ 15/- Rs. (In one year 5 cycles)	Rs. 7,50,000/- (Rs. 1,50,000 per cycle)	Rs. 7,50, 000/-	Rs. 7,50, 000/-	Rs. 7,50, 000/-	Rs. 7,50,00 0/-	Rs. 7,50, 000/-	Rs. 7,50,0 00/-	Rs. 7,50,000/-
2.	Cost of Feeds 3 Kg per bird @ Rs. 18/-	Rs. 27,00,000/- (Rs. 5,40,000/- per cycle)	Rs. 27,00 ,000/-	Rs. 27,00 ,000/-	Rs. 27,00 ,000/-	Rs. 27,00,0 00/-	Rs. 27,00 ,000/-	Rs. 27,00, 000/-	Rs. 27,00,000/ -
3.	Miscellaneous Expenditure (i.e. Electricity, Vaccine, Medicine, Veterianrian	Rs. 2,50,000/- (Rs. 50,000/- per cycle)	Rs. 2,50, 000/-	Rs. 2,50, 000/-	Rs. 2,50, 000/-	Rs. 2,50,00 0/-	Rs. 2,50, 000/-	Rs. 2,50,0 00/-	Rs. 2,50,000/-

	Visit, etc.) Rs. 5/- per bird per batch							
4.	Wages for three labour @ 7000/- per month	Rs. 2,52, 000/-	Rs. 2,52, 000/-	Rs. 2,52, 000/-	Rs. 2,52, 000/-	Rs. 2,52,00 000/-	Rs. 2,52, 000/-	Rs. 2,52, 000/-	Rs. 2,52,000/-
5.	Depreciation on sheds , building etc. @10%	Rs. 2,63, 000/-	Rs. 2,63, 000/-	Rs. 2,63, 000/-	Rs. 2,63, 000/-	Rs. 2,63, 000/-	Rs. 2,63, 000/-	Rs. 2,63, 000/-	Rs. 2,63,000/-
6.	Total Expenditure	Rs. 42,15, 000/-	Rs. 42,15, 000/-	Rs. 42,15, 000/-	Rs. 42,15, 000/-	Rs. 42,15, 000/-	Rs. 42,15, 000/-	Rs. 42,15, 000/-	Rs. 42,15,000/ -

C- INCOME

S.No.	Items	Duration							
		1st Year	2nd Year	3rd Year	4th Year	5th Year	6th Year	7th Year	8th Year
1.	By Broiler Birds Sale @ 60/- Rs. Per Kg for Average 1.8 Kg bird i.e. Rs. 108 on average Rs. 100/- (In one year 5 cycles)	Rs. 47,50,000/- (Rs. 9,50,000 per cycle taken 5% mortality)	Rs. 47,50,0 00/-	Rs. 47,50,0 00/-	Rs. 47,50,0 00/-	Rs. 47,50,0 00/-	Rs. 47,50,0 00/-	Rs. 47,50,0 00/-	Rs. 47,50,0 00/-
2.	By sale of Manure @ Rs. 05/- per Kg	Rs. 5,00,000/- (Rs. 1,00,000/- per cycle)	Rs. 5,00,00 0/-	Rs. 5,00,00 0/-	Rs. 5,00,00 0/-	Rs. 5,00,00 0/-	Rs. 5,00,00 0/-	Rs. 5,00,00 0/-	Rs. 5,00,00 0/-
3.	By sale of Gunny Bags	Rs. 1,00,000/- (Rs. 20,000/- per cycle)	Rs. 1,00,00 0/-	Rs. 1,00,00 0/-	Rs. 1,00,00 0/-	Rs. 1,00,00 0/-	Rs. 1,00,00 0/-	Rs. 1,00,00 0/-	Rs. 1,00,00 0/-
4.	By sale of Equipments and other things after completion of Project	---	---	---	---	---	---	---	Rs. 2,00,00 0/-
5.	Total Income	Rs. 53,50,000/-	Rs. 53,50,0 00/-	Rs. 53,50,0 00/-	Rs. 53,50,0 00/-	Rs. 53,50,0 00/-	Rs. 53,50,0 00/-	Rs. 53,50,0 00/-	Rs. 55,50,0 00/-

D- CALCULATION SHEET

S.No.	Items	Duration							
		1st Year	2nd Year	3rd Year	4th Year	5th Year	6th Year	7th Year	8th Year
1.	Capital Cost	Rs. 26,30,00 0/-	---	---	---	---	---	---	---
2.	Recurring Cost	Rs. 42,15,00 0/-	Rs. 42,15,0 00/-	Rs. 42,15, 000/-	Rs. 42,15,0 00/-	Rs. 42,15,00 0/-	Rs. 42,15,00 0/-	Rs. 42,15,00 0/-	Rs. 42,15,00 0/-
3.	Total Cost	Rs. 68,45,00 0/-	Rs. 42,15,0 00/-	Rs. 42,15, 000/-	Rs. 42,15,0 00/-	Rs. 42,15,00 0/-	Rs. 42,15,00 0/-	Rs. 42,15,00 0/-	Rs. 42,15,00 0/-
4.	Income	Rs. 53,50,00 0/-	Rs. 53,50,0 00/-	Rs. 53,50, 000/-	Rs. 53,50,0 00/-	Rs. 53,50,00 0/-	Rs. 53,50,00 0/-	Rs. 53,50,00 0/-	Rs. 55,50,00 0/-
5.	Net Benefit	Rs. – 14,95,00 0/-	Rs. 11,35,0 00/-	Rs. 11,35, 000/-	Rs. 11,35,0 00/-	Rs. 11,35,00 0/-	Rs. 11,35,00 0/-	Rs. 11,35,00 0/-	Rs. 13,35,00 0/-
6.	Total Benefit	---	---	---	---	---	---	---	Rs. 66,50,00 0/-
7.	Total Benefit per month	---	---	---	---	---	---	---	Rs. 69,271/-

Economics of Layer Farming (30,000 layers)

Salient Features

i) The project report envisages 30000 commercial layer birds to be reared each year.

ii) One brooding batch of 7500 chicks will be reared in Brooder House for 8 weeks.

iii) One growing batch of 7500 chicks will be reared in grower house for 12 weeks.

iv) Four laying batches of 7500 birds i.e. 30000 birds in total will be reared in layer house for 52 weeks.

v) The cost of day old chicks to be purchased & feed has been kept constant for ease incalculation.

vi) The average egg production is considered to be 306 per bird per year.

vii) The average sale price of one egg is assumed Rs. 3.10/-

viii) Birds after 72 weeks of age will be sold @ Rs. 70/- birds for table purpose.

ix) The growing and laying phase mortality is 2 & 3 per cent respectively.

x) 15% extra chicks will be supplied by suppliers.

xi) The brooding, growing phase feed consumption is 0.375 kg and phase feed consumption in laying 0.75 kg per bird per week respectively.

xii) Constructed area for brooder house is taken @ 0.50 sqft. per chick. For grower house 0.60 sqft. Per chick and 0.80 sqft per bird for layer shed.

xiii) The cost of chick, grower and layer feed is kept Rs. 2000, Rs. 1440/- & Rs 1600/- per quintal respectively.

xiv) The term loan from bank will be repayed in seven equal installments starting from next year.

xv) The sale price of empty Gunnybag (bag in which poultry feed is kept) is taken Rs. 20/- each.

xvi) The cost of medicine, vaccine, labour, electricity has been combinedly taken under 10% cost of feed consumed during that year.

Project Summary

The salient features of the project are as:-

i) Total cost of projectis Rs. 180.00/- lac

ii) Bank Loan (70%) Rs. 126.00/- lac

iii) Margin Money (30%) Rs. 54.00/- lac

S.No.	Items	Rate	Rs In lac
·	Land	3 Acres	self
	Building		
B.1	Land Development	-	0.60
B.2	Fencing		1.60
B.3	Brooder shed 3750 sqft	190/-	7.125
B.4	Grower shed 4500 sqft	190/-	8.55
B.5	Layer shed 4x6000=24000 sqft	190/-	45.60
B.6	3000 sqft	190/-	5.70
B.7	Feed Miscellaneous Generator and Equipments		1.125
		Total	**71.25**

	Equipments		
C.1	Brooding equipments for 7500 chicks	50/-	3.75
C.2	Growing equipments for 7500 chicks	70/-	5.25
C.3	Cages for 30000 layers	100/-	30.00
C.4	Automation		1.50
C.5	Water and Electric		3.75
C.6	Feed Mill		6.00
C.7	Weighting Balance		0.75
C.8	Generator		6.75
		Total	**58.50**
	Working Capital		
D.1	Cost of four flocks of 7500 each (4% extra)	27.00	8.10
D.2	Cost of feed for 30000 chicks upto 20 weeks (non productive period)		37.35
D.3	Farm overheads (Medicine, Vaccine, Lab, etc.)		4.20
D.4	Insurance for 4 flocks (30000 birds)	@ Rs 2/bird	0.60
		Total	**50.25**
E	**Cost of the Project**		
a	**Land**		-
b	**Building**		71.25
c	**Equipment & machinery**		58.50
d	**Working capital**		50.25
		Total (E)	**180.00**
	Term loan from bank	70%	126.00
	Margin money	30%	54.00

A. INCOME

1. Sale of eggs and culls

Year	Batch size	No of Batch	Total layer weeks (no)	Prod./bird /year (nos)	Total egg prod (no in lac)	Egg price Rs/ egg	(A) Total sale value Rs in lac	Total culled birds (nos)	(B) From sale of culled birds @Rs 70/- birds	(C) From Sale of Gunny Bags and Manure	Total (A+B+C) Income (Rs. In lac)
I	7500	5	60	306	26.55	3.10	82.29	-	-	2.58	87.54
II	7500	4	216	306	95.98	3.10	296.28	20750	14.50	6.86	317.60
III	7500	5	228	306	100.89	3.10	312.75	34900	24.00	7.00	350.00
IV	7500	4	224	306	99.00	3.10	306.10	27600	19.00	7.00	333.60
V	7500	4	224	306	99.00	3.10	306.10	27600	19.00	7.00	333.60

2. Income from Sale of Gunny Bags and Manure

Year	Batch size	Totalfeed cons. in tones	Total Bags (No)	Price per Bag	Gunny Bag Income Rs. in lac	Manure income Rs.	Total income Rs in Lac (C)
I	30000	546	7800	20	1.58	1.00	2.58
II	30000	1380	19320	20	3.86	3.00	6.86
III	30000	1448	20202	20	4.00	3.00	7.00
IV	30000	1425	19950	20	4.00	3.00	7.00
V	30000	1425	19950	20	4.00	3.00	7.00

B. EXPENDITURE

1. Brooding Phase

Year	Batch size	Brooding weeks	Total feed kgs	Feed cost Rs/Kg	Total Feed cost (Rs in lac)	Medicine Rs 8/ bird (Rs. in lac)	Total Cost (feed+med) (Rs. in lac)
I	30000	8	90000	20.00	18.00	2.40	20.40
II	30000	8	90000	20.00	18.00	2.40	20.40
III	30000	8	90000	20.00	18.00	2.40	20.40
IV	30000	8	90000	20.00	18.00	2.40	20.40
V	30000	8	90000	20.00	18.00	2.40	20.40

2. GrowingPhase

Year	No of Birds	Growing weeks (No)	Feed kg wks/bird	Total feed tones	Feed Cost Rs/kg	Total feed Cost (Rs in lac)	Medicine @Rs 12/- per bird (Rs. In lac)	Total cost (feed+ medicine) Rs.
I	30000	12	0.375	135	14.40	19.44	3.60	23.04
II	30000	12	0.375	135	14.40	19.44	3.60	23.04
III	30000	12	0.375	135	14.40	19.44	3.60	23.04
IV	30000	12	0.375	135	14.40	19.44	3.60	23.04
V	30000	12	0.375	135	14.40	19.44	3.60	23.04

3. Laying Phase

Year	No of Birds Avg. per batch	Laying weeks	Feed kg wk/bird	Total feed tones	Feed Cost Rs/kg	Total Feed Cost (Rs in lac)	medicine cost (Rs. in lac)	Total medi.+ feed cost (Rs in lac)	Total 1+2+3 (Rs in lac)
I	7125	60	0.75	3.20	16.00	51.20	1.50	52.70	96.14
II	7125	216	0.75	11.54	16.00	184.64	3.00	187.64	238.08
III	7125	228	0.75	12.18	16.00	194.88	3.00	197.88	248.32
IV	7125	224	0.75	11.97	16.00	191.52	3.00	194.52	244.96
V	7125	224	0.75	11.97	16.00	191.52	3.00	194.52	244.96

4. Chick Purchase Cost

Year	Batch Size	Total Batches	Total Chicks	Total Cost Rs.
I	7500	5	37500	1012500
II	7500	4	30000	810000
III	7500	5	37500	1012500
IV	7500	4	30000	810000
V	7500	4	30000	810000

C. Salaries Wages and Others

SNo.	Description	No	Salary Per Month	Yearly	Year-II	Year-III	Year-IV	Year-V
1.	Skilled Labour	8	5000	240000	480000	480000	480000	480000
2.	Poultry Attendant	24	3250	512000	876000	876000	876000	876000
3.	Miscellaneous	-	-	48000	48000	48000	48000	48000
	Total			**800000**	**1400000**	**1400000**	**1400000**	**1400000**

D. Annual Income and Expenditure (Rs. lac)

Income	Year					
	I	II	III	IV	V	VI
From sale of egss, culled birds, manure, bags	87.54	317.61	349.80	336.60	333.60	333.60
Expenditure						
Cost of chicks	2.0	8.10	10.125	8.10	8.10	8.10
Cost of Feed, Medicine, Vaccine, etc.	51.20	238.08	248.32	244.96	244.96	244.96
Insurance	-	0.60	0.75	0.60	0.60	0.60
Salary and wages, etc.	3.80	14.00	14.00	14.00	14.00	14.00
Total	**57.00**	**260.78**	**273.22**	**267.66**	**267.66**	**267.66**
Gross Profit	**30.54**	**56.83**	**76.58**	**68.94**	**68.94**	**68.94**
Less Bank Interest	**12.60**	**10.08**	**7.58**	**5.04**	**2.52**	-
Bank Principal	-	**25.20**	**25.20**	**25.20**	**25.20**	**25.20**
Net Saving	**17.94**	**21.55**	**43.80**	**38.70**	**41.22**	**43.74**

Backyard Poultry Production

About 60% rural population in India is depending on agriculture. Poultry has been there in the backyards of most of the houses since ages, forming a part of nutrition and family income. At one time, 30% of the eggs produced were in the backyards. No capital required (only to buy few birds). 5-20 birds can be kept by each household and mainly they are reared to meet the egg and chicken demand of the household. Traditionally they are sold in case of emergency but now these are sold also for income. The birds available for the Backyard farming are less productive for both eggs and meat. Now Central Government, State Government and Non Governmental Organizations (NGO) are mainly concentrating towards Backyard Poultry Farming for better nutrition of poor peoples and their economic upliftment. Central Avian Research Institute (CARI) Bareilly, Central Poultry Development Organization (CPDO), DAHDF, Govt. of India and State Agriculture Universities had developed many breeds for the Backyard farming improving their egg and meat production. Improved varieties "Low technology input birds" are bred for this purpose, which are genetically more efficient in production compared to "Native chicken." The low technology input birds are mostly dual purpose. The birds grow faster than native chicken reaching 1.5 kg weight in 45 days but can withstand variable feed qualities and also supplement themselves by scavenging. The female birds lay 160 eggs against the native birds, which are broody & do not lay more than 60 per year. "Mother Units" are being encouraged to take care of the brooding & vaccination in the early part of growing (first four weeks) before they are distributed. This ensures disease security.

"Cluster farming" in rural areas is possible with these chicken for enhancing the meat production in the lines of broiler farming. A group of 8 to 10 farmers or educated youth can form a cluster and grow the birds in groups of 500 to 1,000 birds in low-cost houses as done in broilers. The birds are grown in "All in All out" basis and the producer works by himself. The group can graduate into "organic chicken" by making their own low-cost feeds without chemicals and antibiotics. The cluster can market the birds in local village mandis or supply them to supermarkets with a brand name. The slow growing multicoloured chicken with tougher meat fetch better price compared to broilers whose meat is tender. This area is developing as a "niche market" with better returns. Brown colour, sturdy layer type birds, laying 300 eggs and more are being considered for "Family Laying Units." States like Kerala have adopted this system as an "alternative system" of egg production to commercial poultry. Even the products are marketed by the farmers directly in weekly village markets and "Collection Centres" established by government or companies.

Poultry Farm Finances

For poultry farming schemes with large outlays Detailed Project Reports (DPR) are required to be prepared. NABARD is the banker of the Banks in Agriculture sector loans i.e. Local Banks provide the loan to the Individual after consent and loan amount from the NABARD. For high value projects, the borrowers can utilise the services of NABARD Consultancy Services (NABCONS), who are having wide experience in preparation of Detailed Project Reports.

Marketing Management

Broiler: Transportation and marketing

Marketing plan should be made in the advance before starting the project. After the birds have been raised to slaughter weight, primarily in open air sheds, they are either bought by the integrators for slaughter and processing, or sold to middle men who sell them on at live markets. In India, marketing is less in the certain festival seasons while demand is more during certain period, that should also be considered while formulating the project. A successful farming depends on the good poultry marketing and good prices. These days Chicken Transportation Crates and Cages are used to transport the broiler, layer or chicks from one place to another without causing any damage. These have excellent ventilation, easy to clean and wash, secure stacking and locking, long life, comfortable and easy to maintain.

Poultry Promotion Schemes and Bankable Project Preparation

Poultry promotion schemes are run by the Central Government i.e. Department of Animal Husbandry, Dairying and Fisheries and State Animal Husbandry Departments. Government agencies are mainly promoting backyard poultry farmers. National Bank for Agriculture and Rural Development (NABARD) helps in the development of Detailed Project Report (DPR) through its technical inputs and it could be contacted on the website https://www.nabard.org/english/home.aspx and detail could be enquired from Nearest Nationalized Bank Branch of the area.

Under development of Poultry Estates, two estates were decided to be established on pilot basis in low commercial activity states / region. Grants were provided to the State Governments for promoting smallholder poultry rearing in rural/tribal areas of the country with refinance from NABARD. Central Poultry Development Organizations have been promoting development of poultry through providing quality chicks for identified low-input technology poultry stocks; diversifying poultry rearing towards duck, turkey & emu, quail and guinea fowl; training of trainers, farmers, women beneficiaries, poultry organizations, NGOs, banks, co-operatives and foreign trainees, etc. and regular testing of various stocks available in the country to assess their performance. Poultry Venture Capital Fund scheme has yielded good result and needs to be continued with thrust on wider publicity and awareness creation among target groups as well as the implementing agencies to derive maximum benefits to diverse stakeholders. Support to rural poultry is also being made available under Swaranjayanti Gram SwarojgarYojana (SGSY) with particular emphasis on group formation of women and the weaker sections. Under Poultry Seed Project being executed by ICAR, rural chicken germplasm is being further improved, multiplied and distributed to various agencies.

□□□

Index

D

E

F

G

H

I

K

L

M

N

O

P

Q

R

S

T

Z

□□□